CARB CYCLING DIET PLAN & COOKBOOK

THE LITTLE CARB CYCLING GUIDE FOR BEGINNERS

CRAIG WILLIAMS

BRITTNEY DAVIS

Cover Design by Rihan W. Cover artwork from DepositPhotos

The Icons used in this work were designed by:

- Freepik, Smashicons, photo3idea_studio, DinosoftLabs, Becris, macrovector, pch.vector, rawpixel.com, vectorpouch, pikisuperstar, Bakar015, Photoroyalty, Terdpongvector, Vextok, Rosapuchalt

Published by Admore Publishing: Berlin, Germany

Printed in the United States of America

www.admorepublishing.com

Disclaimer

This book contains collected information from top experts and sources. All details have been carefully researched and selected but are for informational purposes only. It is not intended to be interpreted as professional medical advice or replace consultation with health care professionals.

Speak to your trusted healthcare professional prior to undergoing any medical procedures, taking any nutritional supplements, or starting an exercise regimen. Reactions and results vary from each individual as there are differences in health conditions.

If you have any underlying health conditions, consult with an appropriately licensed healthcare professional before considering any guidance from this book.

OTHER BOOKS BY BRITTNEY & CRAIG

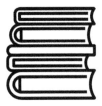

- Liver Detox & Cleanse
- Gut Detox & Cleanse

To find more of our books, simply search or click our names on

www.amazon.com

CONTENTS

FOREWORD

Hi there,

We are Brittney Davis and Craig Williams, and we are passionate about all things health and wellness. Our purpose is to help others in all aspects of building great habits and living a healthier, better life!

You may have grabbed this book because you are interested in finding out more about what carb cycling is and how it can help you lose weight.

Perhaps you are looking for specific recipes and how to easily implement carb cycling in your day to day life...

... Or you are simply on the look for a great way to improve your health and naturally lose weight.

Whatever the reason, **we want to thank you for reading and checking out this book.**

In this book, our aim is to provide a straight-to-the-point, scientifically accurate action plan to getting started with carb cycling. Unlike other health books that focus on overhyped, unhealthy methods to potentially lose weight and detox, we hope to provide you with techniques to improve your wellbeing in a natural form.

Although it's great to read this book all the way through, feel free to skip ahead to different parts you are more interested in. We will cover various topics ranging from the science behind carb cycling and recipes to workout plans and health tips. Skip through topics that may not apply to you and get to the things that may be individually relevant to you!

We sincerely thank you again for your interest. Enjoy!

THE GROUNDWORK OF ALL HAPPINESS IS HEALTH.

Leigh Hunt

AN INTRODUCTION TO CARB CYCLING

It seems like every time you look around, there's a new diet popping up somewhere. First, it was low-fat everything. Then there were the cabbage soup and baby food diets. Then came low-carb, high-protein diets like Atkins, which triggered a backlash against gluten. Then we got keto.

There are more diets out there than there are days of the year, and while some might work, many only work for a while. When you stop eating according to whatever crazy plan it is, every pound comes back, and they all bring a friend!

The basics of losing weight are simple, *in theory*. Burn more calories than you eat. But with our sedentary lifestyles and fast-food culture, that's a lot harder than it seems on paper.

The truth is, most diets are so restrictive or crazy that they are impossible to sustain, and while you might lose a lot of weight on them, the effects are hardly ever long term. Worse, when you do start eating normally again, your body (which thinks it has been starving) tries to store absolutely everything it can. *On your butt.*

Most nutritionists, doctors, and fitness professionals will tell you that diets don't work and that you need to make sustainable lifestyle changes if you want to keep weight off. That's great, but what does that really mean?

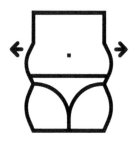

The answer, instead of cutting whole food groups out of your diet, is carb cycling. Which admittedly is a relatively new idea, but it doesn't require you to topple the food pyramid forever! Which is why it's a lot easier to stick to and why your results will last.

If you're reading this, then you're probably at your wit's end. You've probably tried all those weird diets. You probably have a shelf in the bathroom cabinet with pills and potions that didn't work (but cost a fortune), and there's a gym membership in the back of your wallet somewhere. It just hasn't seen the light of day in a while.

The truth is, we do have crazy lives these days. If you're not a celebrity, you're not going to be spending four hours a day getting "ripped," and you can't afford a personal chef to keep your meals healthy all the time.

After eight hours behind a desk, possibly followed by kid wrangling and dog walking, the last thing you want to do is drag yourself to the gym. As for the mornings? Well, when you're burning the candle at both ends, an extra twenty minutes of sleep is a valuable commodity.

The diets have crashed, you can't get yourself to feel the burn, and you're running out of options.

Carb cycling might well be the answer you're looking for. It's not crazy. It doesn't require you to live on lettuce and fat-free everything, and it doesn't require you to buy foods you can't pronounce. It also costs very little, and you can do it without needing a personal trainer and a state-of-the-art treadmill.

That sounds a whole lot better than everything else you've considered, right?

That's what this book is about. I'm going to show you what carb cycling is and the science behind why it works. We're going to look at an effortless way that real people like us can integrate it into our lives, and how to stick to it even when things are a little nuts in your life.

We've even got recipes and a meal plan for you and will show you how fitness (the kind that fits into your life) is so crucial to weight loss in general.

 How do we know that this all works? Because we've been there. We've done the starvation diets, where we felt sick because our stomachs were so empty, and where we felt like we would faint if we stood up too fast. We've tried the diets where you have to throw out everything in your fridge and buy a whole new store cupboard full of things you can't pronounce. We've had the ups, and many of the downs.

Like you, there are days we'd rather be on the couch watching Netflix than outside sweating. But because of carb cycling and some effortless lifestyle changes, we've found a solution that actually works, and that is huge! It's also motivating to see your results pay off, and it's just great to feel healthy.

Diet and exercise shouldn't feel like something you **have to do** with an end goal in sight. It should just be a part of your life, and with this weight loss strategy, it can be.

This book is a guide to making carb cycling work for you. But it's not a magic bullet. Have you ever seen those diet supplement advertisements that say they're "*only effective as part of a healthy diet and exercise plan*", well, that's the trick to everything? It's not the pills or the potions that really get things done. It's eating right and moving more.

This book will show you how to do both, in a safe and healthy way, that won't leave you starving or dreaming about bread. The weight loss on a plan like this is not as dramatic in the short term, admittedly, but it's infinitely more sustainable. As with everything, however, all of the parts of the carb cycling plan are important, and you need to balance your eating plan with activity. Fortunately, that's not nearly as hard to do as some other plans are!

So, if you're ready to get off the crash diet hamster wheel and find a healthy weight loss option that actually works long term, read on. This book was written for you.

YOUR GOALS, MINUS YOUR DOUBTS, EQUAL YOUR REALITY.

Ralph Marston

1

WHAT IS CARB CYCLING?

If you feel like there's a new weight-loss fad every other day, you're probably not far off. Ever since we realized that being a healthy weight was better for us, and since skinny became the pinnacle of beauty in most fashion magazines and on runways worldwide, people everywhere have been looking for quick fixes and weight loss hacks.

It's not just women either. Men and women around the world are looking for ways to lose weight, across all age groups, backgrounds, and races. In fact, studies have shown that as many as 45 million Americans are dieting every year. That's about 13% of the population!

We all want tighter abdominal muscles, tauter butts, bigger muscles, or slimmer hips. Still, most of those diet crazes won't deliver these results, or at least, not for long.

Carb cycling may sound like just another weight loss buzzword, especially if you're already exhausted from counting calories, reading food labels, and burning all the processed food in your home. But unlike most of the diets out there, there's some real science behind this weight-loss method, and more and more people are showing remarkable, sustainable results.

In this chapter, we're looking at the nuts and bolts of carb cycling. What it is, where it came from, how and why it works, and what you can expect as you get started.

What Is Carb Cycling

Carb cycling is an eating plan that is based on the idea of alternating between high carb and low carb days. Unlike cutting out carbs completely, that tends to leave people suffering from actual, physical withdrawal symptoms and crazy cravings. This allows people who follow the diet to get some carbs but not overwhelm their bodies with too many.

Since we already know that our western diets generally just have too much of everything, that already sounds like a better plan. Just from a moderation point of view, but there are some genuine scientific reasons for why this works.

In fact, carb cycling has been around for a while, in professional sports, and amongst aspiring athletes. If these top athletes, who have coaches, nutritionists, and sports doctors working to get them in peak physical condition (and keep them there), trust this method, then we're definitely on to a good thing.

The Science of Carb Cycling

One of the reasons our modern, sedentary lifestyles have caused us to get out of shape is that our bodies, by design, don't like routine.

That's why personal trainers recommend changing the type of exercise you do to get the best results. It's also why, when you are stuck in a diet and exercise rut, your basal metabolic rate (or the rate at which you metabolize food) drops right to the floor.

Our bodies need variety, whether in high-intensity interval training or exercising different muscle groups on different days and mixing cardio with strength training. So, variety really is *the spice of life*, but there are some excellent reasons for that.

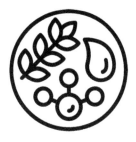

When you eat food that contains a lot of carbohydrates, your blood sugar goes up, and that signals your pancreas to make more insulin to transport glucose to your cells. Your cells then either burn that glucose as energy, store it for a short time, or convert it into fat for long term storage.

As your cells are taking in glucose, your pancreas also tells your cells to release the stored form of glucose, called glucagon. This helps keep your blood sugar levels in balance, your cells fuelled, and gives you the energy you need to live.

The problem with all of this comes into play when you make too much insulin, because you're consuming too many carbs. This causes your cells to store more glucose, convert more into fat, and can lead to type 2 diabetes or heart disease.

Carb cycling reduces the amount of carbs you consume on certain days. This means that instead of excess glucose to use as fuel, cells are forced to burn stored fat, which results in weight loss, and lower overall body fat.

This process works best when you are also working out at least moderately most days (particularly on high carb days), so that you burn most of the energy from the carbs you do eat. It also means that you may still gain weight or not lose enough weight if you don't exercise because of the high carb days.

So there's a careful balance of science and practical considerations involved in carb cycling. Still, most doctors and fitness experts agree that, at least in the short term, it's a good, safe way to lose weight without starving yourself, and is likely to result in sustainable results.

Carb Cycling Basics

The science behind carb cycling is proven, reasonably simple to understand, and based on real-world evidence. So, how do you make it work for you?

Individual plans will vary based on your current weight, desired weight loss, and fitness and activity levels. Still, the general plan for carb cycling is to alternate high carb days with low carb days.

For instance, your high carb days may include, for example, 175 grams of carbs, and low carb days would be 100 grams. If you were just alternating between high carb and low carb days, you might start with a high carb day on Monday, low carb on Tuesday, high carb on Wednesday, and so on.

If you were looking to lose more weight, or are want faster results, the amount of carbs you consume on each low and high day might be reduced, and if you really want to kickstart your weight loss, you might even add a "no-carb day" into the cycle.

It's important to note that when this plan talks about carbs, it's not about highly processed, highly sugared and salted snacks, along with refined white bread or rice. The carbs you choose for your carb cycling eating plan should be high quality, fiber-rich options like brown rice, sweet potatoes, and so on.

Even if you have "permission" to eat carbs, highly processed foods have little nutritional value and extremely high caloric content. This defeats the whole purpose of even attempting to begin a healthier eating plan.

Who Can Implement Carb Cycling?

Carb cycling is suitable for most people. Actually, it's even good for most people because it helps control blood sugar and insulin levels.

Carb cycling is commonly used by professional and high-level athletes, but even people who have demanding physical jobs or lifestyles can use carb cycling to control their weight. Since it doesn't require any special foods or supplements, there's also no high financial cost to get started. Although it's a simple way to get started on your weight-loss journey, anytime you plan to make any lifestyle changes, including diet or exercise, you should always consult your doctor for guidance and advice. Not only will your doctor be able to give you the "*all clear*," but they might also be able to offer resources and information that will help you get started.

However, it should be noted that people who have complex relationships with food and eating disorders should be cautious about getting started with this eating plan. It requires a high level of monitoring and control, which can potentially be a negative trigger for some with unhealthy eating conditions. If you have suffered from an eating disorder and you want to try carb cycling, you should first speak to your counselor, therapist, or mental health professional, to ensure that you can do it safely and healthily.

Other people who should avoid carb cycling or only try it under their doctors' advice and direction are pregnant women, women who are breastfeeding, and people who are already at their ideal weight or underweight.

Shifting Those Last Stubborn Pounds

Often, people who have larger amounts of weight to lose find that their weight loss starts out well by merely changing what types of food they eat and how much of it they consume. This is then multiplied by adding some exercise to their routine.

However, as your weight loss continues towards your goal weight, you might start to notice that your losses slow down considerably. In fact, most people find that the last ten to fifteen pounds are the hardest to shift.

Remember how we mentioned that your body gets into a rut, gets comfortable, and effectively stops or slows your weight loss down? That's precisely what happens, even if you're doing everything right.

So, if you've found that your weight loss has stalled, but you're still doing everything you're supposed to, carb cycling can be the boost you need to get things moving again.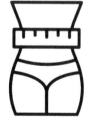

Carb cycling can also be a good thing to do periodically when you notice that your weight is edging a little in the wrong direction, for the same reason.

Carb Cycling for Athletes

Carb cycling isn't only for people who are looking to lose weight. It's also for people who are already living healthy lifestyles. Those who want to build muscle mass, lose bodyweight, or store more carbs for an event like a marathon.

However, in those cases, because they have very specific goals that are directly related to their performance in their sport of choice, it's almost always advisable that they seek a nutritionist or dietician's advice.

While most of us can make adjustments to our diet without impacting our performance in our lives or in our jobs or without too much other trouble, even small changes to your diet might have a profound effect if you are competing in a sport.

Since athletes also need to be more careful balancing lean proteins with carbs and other nutrients, it's a lot trickier to get everything exactly right at this level.

Side Effects of Carb Cycling

Carb cycling works, and it's safe for most people, but that doesn't mean that making changes to your diet won't have some sort of side effects. If you've ever tried to quit sugar or cut back on coffee, you know that changes in your diet can have physical and mental effects for a while, as you get used to the new normal.

Fortunately, these side effects are relatively mild and are short-lived. They might include:

- Changes in sleep patterns.
- General tiredness or slight fatigue.

- Gastrointestinal issues like constipation or bloating.
- Mood changes.

These symptoms frequently occur when people change their carbohydrate intake and are much more severe when cutting carbs out completely. It's so common, it's known as "carb flu," and it usually subsides once your body adjusts to your new diet, generally in a few days to a week.

One of the Simpler Diet Plans

As you can see, there's nothing overly complicated about carb cycling. Because you still get to have some carbs, it's much less restrictive than many other diets.

While you still need to maintain a healthy caloric intake for your body type, age, gender, and weight loss goals, you have quite a lot of leeway regarding dietary choices. You also won't need to invest a small fortune in obscure foods and expensive supplements.

Now that we've looked at the basics, the science, and the health considerations you need to make, it's time to get into specifics about what you can eat, when you can eat it, and how to plan your carb cycling journey.

IF YOU KEEP GOOD FOOD IN YOUR FRIDGE, YOU WILL EAT GOOD FOOD.

Errick McAdams

2

THE DIET

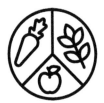

You are what you eat. Much more so than you think.

I used to be quite the couch potato who enjoyed eating plenty of soft white bread, and you guessed it. I definitely looked a little doughy before making positive changes to my habits. Even though this is general knowledge, it's still challenging to make the adjustments we know we need to make.

Especially when the diet you're following is complicated and far outside of the norm.

Carb cycling isn't like that. It doesn't require you to learn to love foods you can't pronounce and shop at overpriced organic markets. You can still eat regular foods – just with a few simple changes.

In this chapter, we're going to look at the diet aspect of carb cycling in more detail. We're going to look at specific foods that are a good idea and some that you should limit. We're also going to take a closer look at the nutrients that make up our diets, what they do, and why we need them.

Because that's key to understanding why restrictive diets are a bad idea. Eliminating anything is not a good idea. But limiting, moderating, and controlling what, when, and how we eat, makes all the difference.

The Diet

As we've already mentioned, carb cycling doesn't work if you don't exercise while controlling your carb intake. Still, since the exercise required to make it work is moderate and not exactly going to throw your lifestyle into chaos, we're going to start with the diet.

You may be familiar with the 80/20 rule for diet and exercise. It's hard to believe for many, but there is a lopsided balance of importance when it comes to the gym versus the kitchen. The best health and fitness results are determined mostly by the food you eat (80%) and only minimally by your workouts (20%). Working out is essential and brings a host of benefits besides looking and feeling good, but it definitely pays to pay close attention to your nutrition.

Nutrition

All good diet plans are built around healthy nutrition. No matter how much we want to look better, it doesn't matter if we aren't healthy. You can be just as unhealthy starving yourself to be "skinny" as you can if you are overweight. It all comes down to nutrients.

Our bodies need various components in the foods we eat to perform specific functions, and if we don't get them, we will not be healthy. It is that simple.

Carbohydrates, Proteins, and Fats

Over the last few years, diet gurus have really changed the way we look at food. Where low fat and counting calories was all the rage in the 1980s, the late 1990s brought a new trend that convinced us that carbohydrates were the root of all evil. Some diet gurus even went as far as recommending to eat as much fat and protein as possible.

Today, what we now know about healthy diets is that carbohydrates aren't evil, and neither is fat. Protein is not a magical weight-loss elixir, and it's more important to balance what we eat and eat the right kinds of all of those things. Here's what you need to know.

Carbohydrates

Carbohydrates are further divided into starch, sugar, and fiber. They're found in foods like grains, grain products, fruits, and vegetables. While they have had a bad reputation for a while, they're not inherently bad. In fact, because carbohydrates give our cells the quick, easily accessible energy they need, they are absolutely essential to our health.

Carbohydrates are named for their chemical structure, which is simply carbon, hydrogen, and oxygen.

The average carbohydrate goal for adults is around 135 grams per day. However, this varies per person, and it's recommended that about 45 to 65% of your diet is made up of carbohydrates.

Aside from providing an easy and readily available source of energy for your body, carbs are also crucial for brain function and even for stabilizing your mood. In fact, the recommended daily allowance of carbs takes not only your body's energy needs into account but also the amount of carbs your brain needs to function.

Proteins

Proteins are called the building blocks of the body because they are. All of our cells, tissues, and even bones are made from protein. It is also the basis of many of the chemicals and enzymes in our body. In particular, hemoglobin is a vital protein, which carries oxygen around the body.

In short, we cannot exist without protein.

At any given time, there are more than 10,000 proteins at work in your body.

But even though protein is so important, there are an increasing number of studies that show that people in the developed world eat far more protein than they need. Like everything else, this is a case of too much of a good thing being bad for you.

To use proteins, our bodies either break them down into their building blocks, known as amino acids or modified amino acids, to make different ones. There are, however, nine amino acids that our body cannot produce from others. These are known as essential amino acids, and they include:

- Isoleucine
- Histidine
- Valine

- Leucine
- Lysine
- Methionine
- Phenylalanine
- Threonine
- Tryptophan

We need all of these amino acids to be healthy, which means we need various protein-rich foods to get everything we need.

The good news is that we don't need much protein to get all the amino acids we need. In fact, we only need about 0.35 grams of protein for every pound of body weight, so if you weigh 200 lbs, you only need about 70 grams of protein to be healthy! If your goal is to build muscle, you will definitely need more than this minimum value. However, your body is already able to function correctly with these small amounts.

Most of our western diets actually include far too much protein.

It's also important to note that the source of your protein matters. Choose lean, unprocessed meat, poultry, and fish, rather than processed, salt and nitrate heavy processed meats. You can also get protein from eggs, dairy products, and vegetable sources like beans and other legumes.

Wherever you get your protein, make sure it's high quality, and remember that a little goes a long way!

Fats

Fat has a bad reputation. But it's really just as necessary as carbs and protein in a healthy diet. In fact, certain fatty acids are essential for things like brain function. Without them, your brain simply cannot function properly. Even babies need fat in their diet so that their brains can develop properly.

Fats also help with nerve function and nutrient absorption. Like protein, there are some types of fatty acids that you can't manufacture yourself and have to get from food. Those are known as essential fatty acids.

Most healthy people need between 30 and 45 milliliters of fat per day, which is between two and three tablespoons – so definitely not a lot! It's also important to remember that the type of fats matter. Unsaturated fats, which are usually from plant-based sources and are generally liquid at room temperature, like olive oil, are good for you. Animal fats, which are also known as saturated fats, and are usually solid at room temperature, are not. Saturated fats are the kind that clog arteries and cause heart conditions!

Other essential fats to choose are Omega 3, 6, and 9, which we get from nuts, seeds, canola oil, fatty fish, and similar sources.

Despite everything you've heard about choosing low fat, healthy fats are not only okay to eat, but they're also necessary to stay healthy. Added bonus? Foods that contain healthy fats like nuts or full-fat dairy products tend to leave us feeling fuller for longer, so they're a great choice in moderation.

While trans fat is present naturally in some dairy and meat products, it's not a healthy choice when it is a manufactured part of processed foods. You should already be limiting processed food consumption, but you should definitely take everything that contains trans fats off your grocery list!

Simple Versus Complex Carbs

Many people think that people who have diabetes only have to avoid sugar, but that's not true. In fact, diabetics have to be incredibly careful about the quantity and type of carbs they eat as well, because carbohydrates cause blood sugar levels to rise.

But carbs aren't created equal. While some types of carbs cause a rapid spike in blood sugar and then an equally rapid drop, others are more reliable, causing a slower rise and drop in energy levels.

Complex carbohydrates are carbs that contain more prolonged and more complex chains of sugars, which take longer to break down into glucose. This includes foods like bread and pasta.

Simple carbohydrates contain simple sugars, like table sugar and syrup. There's extraordinarily little time between when you eat simple carbohydrates and when the glucose is released into your blood. This is what we know as a sugar rush – a spike of sugar in the blood, followed by a sharp drop.

Of course, because carb cycling is based on the idea of encouraging cells to release sugars slower, store fewer carbs and burn fat for energy, it's always preferable to choose complex carbs when possible.

Some healthy foods like dairy products, fruit, and similar do also contain simple sugars. So when you eat those types of foods, it's a good idea to choose higher fiber options (like a piece of fruit instead of fruit juice) and combine it with some fat and protein. This helps slow down digestion (like an apple and a bit of cheese as a snack.)

As always, when you are choosing the carbs you plan to eat, opt for less refined products over white flour, sugar, or rice. Brown rice, whole grains, and whole fruits are always better for you than their processed counterparts.

Macronutrients

Our diet, whatever it may be, is made up of macronutrients and micronutrients.

The word macro means large, and that's what this type of nutrient is – a large, high-level group of food types. This includes carbohydrates, fats, protein, and so on.

Micro means small, and that's what those nutrients are – smaller building blocks of the foods we eat. These include vitamins, minerals, amino acids, and trace elements that we need to stay healthy.

A healthy, balanced diet will have enough of both of these types of nutrients in the proper ratios. If you get that right, then the actual foods you choose are less of a problem.

Food Guidelines

Before you can make the changes necessary to make carb cycling work for you, you first need to know what a healthy diet looks like.

Things have changed a little in recent years too. We've discovered that carbs might be less of a problem than we once thought, but also that sugar might be far more harmful than we believed. Since sugar is commonly added to low-fat foods, and since we have also learned that low-fat products aren't always better for us and that fat is not inherently bad, that's changed a lot about what we define as healthy eating. Here are the basic rules for healthy eating you need to know:

- Imagine that each plate of food you eat is divided into fractions.
- About half of the plate should be made up of fruits and vegetables.
- A quarter of the plate should be healthy, lean proteins.
- The final quarter should be whole grains and wholegrain products.
- Try to cook your own meals as much as possible. This allows you to control precisely what you eat.
- Eat slower and enjoy your food. Use herbs, spices, and similar flavorings to make your food tastier.
- Always read food labels and avoid foods that are highly processed or contain a lot of preservatives.
- Whenever possible, shop from the outer isles or ring of the supermarket. This is usually where the healthy, fresh foods are kept!
- Whenever possible, choose water as your beverage of choice.

It's also worth remembering that if you're eating healthy most of the time, you can have the occasional treat. Use the 90/10 rule to determine your eating choices. If you eat healthy 90% of the time, you can treat yourself 10% of the time.

While you might think that treats are taboo, people tend to crave things they can't have. If you ban anything from your diet outright, you're only going to want it more. So, have it occasionally, in moderation.

What Carbs Do

Carbohydrates, as we have already established, are our body's primary energy source. But it's what we use that energy for that makes them essential.

Fiber, which is a carbohydrate, helps your digestive system function properly, makes you feel fuller for longer, and helps keep your cholesterol in check.

They help your brain and central nervous system function properly, which keeps all of your other systems working properly. They also help organs and systems like your kidneys and liver perform their functions.

Your cells and muscles also store carbohydrates, so when you are working out or doing a strenuous activity, they have energy available to fuel you. That's why athletes "carbo-load." They need the stored energy from carbs to keep them going during marathons and similar endurance tests.

The Problem with Excess Carbs

We already know that as citizens of the modern world, where we have an abundance of food available all the time, we really eat too much of everything. Too much sugar, too much fat, too much protein, and too many carbs. All of those things can be bad for you.

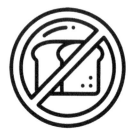

It's important to note again that carbs themselves aren't bad. They're not the dietary bogeyman, and we all need them to be healthy. But we need them in the right quantities.

When you eat too many carbs, and especially if they are the wrong type of carbs, you will experience several unwanted side effects.

Too many carbs will cause your blood sugar to spike. That, in turn, triggers your pancreas to create more insulin, and more insulin tells your cells to store the extra carbs as fat. If this cycle continues, it can lead to permanent problems like Type 2 diabetes.

Because carbs are fuel, we only need enough to fuel the processes our body performs. The less we do, the fewer carbs we need to eat.

Stabilizing Blood Sugar and Losing Fat

If you've always been a calorie counter when it comes to weight loss, then you might be surprised to find that while calories are important, it's actually equally important to keep your blood sugar stable. As we previously mentioned, when your blood sugar spikes, it triggers a chain reaction that ends with carbs being stored as fat.

If you continue to eat more carbs than you need, you will keep storing them as fat, and you will never use the fat reserves you already have as energy instead. Over time, this results in excess fat deposits and weight gain, and it becomes a self-perpetuating cycle.

The critical thing to remember here is that you do still need carbs – so you just have to control the amount you eat and the type of carbs you choose. Of course, refined carbs combined with fat and sugar (*yes, we're talking to you doughnuts*) are not a great choice!

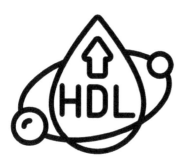

Because carb cycling controls the amount of carbs you eat and gives you days where you eat a little less than you need, your blood sugar stays stable most days. This allows your cells to have the opportunity to tap into those fat stores.

Boosting Clarity, Focus, and Energy

When we think about burning energy, our thoughts immediately go to exercise and physical energy. That's not wrong – we do need more energy if we're more active. But that's not the only thing that requires energy.

Everything your body does, including thinking, requires energy, and when you are starved of carbs, you don't have that. That's why people who cut out carbs entirely have headaches, mood swings, and mental fog.

Believe it or not, your brain uses about 20% of the energy your body uses in total in a day. So you literally need carbs to think properly!

Caloric Deficit for Fat Loss

There's a very old and very simple equation for losing weight:

Energy required > energy consumed = weight loss

That's true. No matter what diet you are on, whether you are limiting calories to see fast results, cutting out food groups, or counting calories on a traditional diet.

Carb cycling combines all of the best tactics into one eating plan that's easier to sustain. Calories are limited to recommended levels, but because there are some days with more carbs and some with less, each day may be different.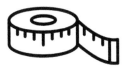

Because people who choose carb cycling aren't cutting out whole food groups, they don't tend to have intense cravings for things that are bad for them, which means less chance of binge eating. It also means that they won't be deficient in macro or micronutrients.

Also, because you are still eating carbs when cycling, you won't have the adverse effects of low or no-carb diets, like headaches and brain fog.

The truth is, creating a caloric deficit is the only sure-fire way to guarantee weight loss, but that doesn't mean it's easy to sustain. Carb cycling eliminates some of the problems with this approach, by spreading the effects over time rather than requiring you to make drastic changes every day.

If you can stick to a diet that includes a caloric deficit over time, the only possible outcome is weight loss. It's really that simple.

Life Is for Living, Not Deprivation

Perhaps the most important argument for carb cycling is that you don't have to cut out anything you really love. This is why most diets fail. They require you to deprive yourself of things you love to eat, and while most people can do that in the short term, it becomes harder and harder over time.

Carb cycling still allows you to enjoy foods you love, especially on high carb days. This makes low carb days much easier to handle, since you know you only have one day to wait to enjoy some of those foods again.

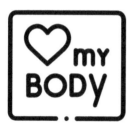

Diet, health, and exercise are essential, but we should always remember why we want to be healthy – so we can enjoy a longer life. And the key word here is **enjoy**. If you can never eat things you love or indulge in take-out, or anything else, your life will be a very grey and boring existence.

Because carb cycling doesn't make you choose enjoyment over weight loss, you're far more likely to stick with it for the longer term. Its consistency that really helps you to lose weight healthily and naturally.

Organizing the Plan

Ever heard the saying, "*failing to plan is planning to fail*"? That's true for everything in life, and weight loss is no different. Whatever you want to do in life, whether it's losing weight, training for a marathon, quitting smoking, or something else, you are much more likely to succeed if you plan before you leap right in.

So, while you might be super excited to jump right in, take a breath, and take a moment to plan for success!

· · ·

Carb Cycling for Beginners

If you are new to carb cycling and to carb restrictive diets, then you probably don't want to leap right into a super intense plan. This can give you "carb flu," make you feel terrible, and causes you to quit before you even start to see results.

It's always best to ease into diet and lifestyle changes, so you don't shock your system and experience those kinds of negative results.

So if you are doing this for the first time, you probably want to opt for a simple plan with four days of low carbs and three days of high carbs per week, alternating between the two.

Easing into carb cycling like this should help you to avoid any dramatic side effects and limit cravings related to cutting back on carbs on certain days.

Advanced Carb Cycling

Once you get used to carb cycling and are used to eating fewer carbs on certain days of the week, you can move to a more advanced plan with five or six days of low carb eating and 1 to 2 days of higher carb eating.

While this is more intense and requires more will power, it will also offer faster weight loss results, so it may be an attractive option.

It's important to note that you don't have to stay on either of these plans all the time. You can always switch between the two when you feel you need to increase or decrease the intensity of your eating plan.

. . .

Determine Intake Levels

There's no hard and fast rule that puts a single figure on how many carbs you should be eating when you are carb cycling. Most of it is subjective and based on individual needs. However, there are a few rules you can follow to get started.

Your Daily Calorie Limit or Goal

The first thing you need to do when you start planning carb cycling is to determine (if you don't already know it) what your total daily calorie intake should be. This will depend on various factors and may require a visit to a doctor, nutritionist, or fitness and weight loss specialist to determine, but there are a few basic rules of thumb:

- For the average woman who is not trying to lose weight and just wants to maintain her weight, the average caloric intake is about 2,000 calories per day.
- If you are a woman and want to lose weight at a rate of 1lb per week, you need to reduce that to about 1,500 calories per day.
- Men who want to maintain their weight can eat about 2,500 calories per day.

- Men who want to lose weight slowly should reduce that to about 2,000 calories per day.

Keep in mind, your height, starting weight, age, fitness and activity level, metabolism, and many other factors also play a role here. So these numbers may vary based on your unique situation.

You can use two basic methods to determine your average caloric intake keeping you at your current weight. This is what is considered your "maintenance" calories as it describes the number of calories needed to *maintain* you at your current level.

The first method uses the Harris-Benedict equation. This equation is widely regarded as one of the more accurate ways of determining someone's maintenance calories. It is the most well-known equation, and although it has been revised twice, it still produces very similar results to what was pointed out already in 1918. The latest revision, which we describe in detail below, takes into account your BMR (basal metabolic rate) and considers your lifestyle, be it highly active or inactive.

It may come as a surprise, but your body is actually burning calories all the time. Even when you do nothing, your body continuously works on things you are unconscious of, such as pumping blood through your body, digestion, and breaking down nutrients. This work burns the majority (70%) of the calories you use daily and is called your BMR.

Your BMR can be calculated as follows:

CALCULATING BMR FOR WOMEN

Harris-Benedict Formula revised by Mifflin - St. Joer

IMPERIAL

(4.536 × weight in lb) + (15.88 × height in inches) – (5 × age) – 161 = BMR

METRIC

(10 × weight in kg) + (6.25 × height in cm) – (5 × age in years) – 161 = BMR

EXAMPLE

A woman who weighs 170 pounds, is 5 feet 5 inches tall, and is 30 years old would have a BMR of 1,492.

CALCULATING BMR FOR MEN

Harris-Benedict Formula revised by Mifflin - St. Joer

IMPERIAL

(4.536 × weight in lb) + (15.88 × height in inches) – (5 × age) + 5 = BMR

METRIC

(10 × weight in kg) + (6.25 × height in cm) – (5 × age in years) + 5 = BMR

EXAMPLE

A man who weighs 200 pounds, is 5 feet 10 inches tall, and is 30 years old would have a BMR of 1,873.

The next step is to combine this information with your lifestyle. The number of calories you need will differ depending on how active you are. The Harris-Benedict equation takes this information into consideration by splitting up how active you may be into 5 categories:

- Sedentary: In this case, you would be performing very little or no exercise at all. *BMR x 1.2*
- Lightly Active: In this case, you would be performing some exercise, 1 to 3 times per week. *BMR x 1.375*
- Moderately Active: In this case, you would perform a moderate amount of exercise, 3 to 5 times per week. *BMR x 1.55*
- Highly Active: In this case, you are very active and work out 6 to 7 times per week. *BMR x 1.725*
- Extremely Active: In this case, you work out multiple times a day or exercise daily, and work a highly physical job. *BMR x 1.9*

Examples: The woman and man described in the BMR calculation working office jobs and performing no exercise would have the following maintenance calories.

Woman: 1,790 calories per day

Man: 2,248 calories per day

This is a great way to get started and can give you relatively accurate figures. However, the equation can still have errors. The formula does not take into account body composition and metabolism. According to the equation, a person who has a higher amount of muscle yet weighs the same as an overweight individual will have the same maintenance calories. However, this would be incorrect as muscle and fat require a different amount of calories for maintenance. The formula has also been tested on hundreds of thousands of people, giving an excellent general result. It does not, though, provide a figure precisely for you.

This brings us to the second method to determine your maintenance calories. It will require you to keep track of the calories you consume for at least a week, preferably two weeks. Overall our bodies are relatively good at keeping us at a consistent weight and telling us what it needs. If you find yourself very hungry, it is commonly because you haven't eaten in a while or burned many calories from a workout the day before. If you don't feel hungry on a day, it can be because you had some large meals the day before. Although the number of calories you consume may vary from day to day, you will find your average maintenance calories over the long run (2 weeks of tracking).

An example of an average man's caloric intake for a week is as follows:

Day 1 - 2400 calories

Day 2 - 2700 calories

Day 3 - 1900 calories

Day 4 - 3200 calories

Day 5 - 2070 calories

Day 6 - 3400 calories

Day 7 - 2600 calories

Average: 2610

After 7 days, this individual can estimate that their maintenance calories are around 2600 calories. Tracking for 14 days will give an even more complete picture. Still, an average of 7 days can already show an accurate estimate.

Losing Weight

Now that we understand how many calories we are consuming to maintain our weight, it becomes a lot easier to see how we can successfully lose weight. If your goal is to lose weight, it's great to cut your maintenance calories by 500 calories per day. For example, if you find your maintenance calories are around 2600 calories per day, reduce your caloric intake to 2100 calories per day. This caloric deficit can either be achieved by reducing the number of calories you eat or through the combination of eating less and doing more.

Calculating High Carb Day Requirements

Once you know how many calories you need to consume each day, the next step is to figure out what proportion of that should be carbs.

The average person who does not control their carb intake needs to get about 60% of their daily nutrition from complex carbs. This will be the amount for your "high carb" days, so you can calculate the number of calories from carbs as follows:

Daily calories x 60% = Calories from complex carbs

The rest of your calories will come from protein, fat, dairy products, and so on. Remember that carbs include fruits and vegetables, too, because carbs can be sugars, starch, or fiber. So, the 60% you will be eating will be fruits, vegetables, grains, etc.

Calculating Low Carb Day Requirements

Most doctors and nutritionists agree that "ketosis," which is when your body stops burning carbs as fuel and moves on to fat (which is the goal for any weight loss plan!), happens when you consume about 50 grams of carbs per day.

If you want to use that as your carb goal for the day, you will definitely be in the right range. Still, there is another potential option if this is too harsh of a change for beginners. You can start by halving your high carb daily allowance. Alternatively, some doctors even recommend having carb cycles that increase from 50 grams to 100 grams, then 150 grams and 200 grams, and then back to 50 grams. That's a more gradual way of doing things, but it should mean you have less of a "shock to your system" when you go from high carb to low carb days!

Different Goal - Different Strategies

One of the advantages of implementing carb cycling to achieving your health goals is that it is very flexible. You can tweak almost anything to make it fit into your schedule and have it work for you. This flexibility is also what makes it one of the more complicated strategies to execute for beginners. When starting out, you simply want to be told what to do and have it work. Below we have laid out 2 guidelines for beginners to follow depending on whether the goal is to lose weight or gain muscle.

.   .   .

Goal: Weight Loss

As we previously laid out, when it comes to weight loss, it's all about calories in versus calories out. If you consistently burn more calories than you consume, you will lose weight. Now, we also learned, and many of us have also experienced, that although this sounds easy, it can be highly challenging. Below are some example carb cycling plans that can help you achieve your weight loss goals. There is no best option as they are all effective, and it's up to you to follow the one you prefer (A, B, or C).

CARB CYCLING FOR WEIGHT LOSS

	OPTION A	OPTION B	OPTION C
MON	Low Carb	Low Carb	Low Carb
TUES	High Carb	Low Carb	Medium Carb
WED	Low Carb	High Carb	High Carb
THURS	High Carb	Low Carb	Low Carb
FRI	Low Carb	Low Carb	Medium Carb
SAT	High Carb	Low Carb	High Carb
SUN	Low Carb	High Carb	Low Carb

Low Carb & Medium Carb: Aim for a deficit of 500 calories and a maximum of 50-100 grams of carbs.

High Carb: Aim for a deficit of 250 calories and getting up to 60% of your calories from carbs.

Goal: *Gain Muscle*

For those looking to gain some weight in muscle, carb cycling can be an effective strategy. It will allow you to increase muscle mass in a controlled manner without potentially also gaining lots of fat. The important thing here is to perform lots of strength training (5-6 times per week). This increased strength training, along with consuming an adequate amount of protein, will lead to gaining the right kind of weight. Aim to consume 1 gram of protein per pound of bodyweight. So if you weigh 200 pounds, you will want to eat 200 grams of protein daily. Below are some example carb cycling plans that can help gain muscle.

CARB CYCLING FOR GAINING MUSCLE

	OPTION A	OPTION B	OPTION C
MON	High Carb	High Carb	High Carb
TUES	Low Carb	High Carb	Medium Carb
WED	High Carb	Low Carb	Low Carb
THURS	Low Carb	High Carb	High Carb
FRI	High Carb	High Carb	Medium Carb
SAT	Low Carb	Low Carb	Low Carb
SUN	High Carb	High Carb	High Carb

High Carb: Aim for a surplus of maximum 250 calories and getting up to 60% of your calories from carbs. Aim for 1 gram of protein per pound of bodyweight.

Low Carb & Medium Carb: Aim for a surplus of 250 calories and a maximum of 50-100 grams of carbs. Maintian 1 gram of proterin per pound of your bodyweight.

In Combination with Exercise

We will dive deeper into the importance of exercise throughout Chapter 12. Still, we wanted to already describe a bit of the relationship between exercise and carb cycling. Now that you have decided on a carb cycling strategy dependent on your goal (losing weight or gaining muscle), where does working out fit in?

It's quite simple, on the days you consume more carbs, that's when you want to get a good workout in. The higher amount of carbs will give you more energy and allow you to power through exercises. The exercise you perform is up to you and what your goals are. Make sure it is something you enjoy doing, this way, it will be easier for you to stick to it.

On your low carb days, you can take it a bit easier. If you are motivated, you can nevertheless do some exercise as it won't hurt your progress. Still, you may find yourself a little lower on energy and not able to perform at your highest level. These days are great to go for a nice walk, do some stretching, and prepare for a big workout coming up on a high carb day.

Monitor and Adjust

Most people will find that they don't hit the carb cycling "sweet spot" on their first try. You may find that you're not getting results fast enough. Or maybe you have unpleasant side effects from drastically reduced carbs on your low carb days. Also, although online calculators can help generate esti- 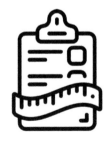 mates for your daily calorie limit and some calculating the proteins, fats, and carbs you should consume, it is essential to realize these are estimates. Unless you have access to highly accurate calory trackers or a nutritionist, you will need to do a bit of experimenting and monitoring.

Take careful note of how you feel and how your weight loss is going for a week or two, and then adjust the values for low and high carb days accordingly. Just don't go below 50 grams of carbs without talking to a doctor or nutritional expert. You do still need some carbs in your diet every day to be healthy!

Preparing for Success

No matter what you're planning to do, planning ahead, getting into the right mindset, and being entirely sure you're ready to commit is a big part of the success of any life change.

Contrary to what you might have been told, science says that it takes the average person about 66 days (not 21!) to really embrace a new habit. This is the point where it becomes automatic.

So, if you want to make carb cycling a part of your lifestyle, you're going to need to commit to at least two months before it becomes a part of your routine. Making the necessary preparations to make it easy to do during that period will make sticking to your new eating plan for two months a lot easier.

Grocery Shopping

When you are trying to change your diet, there's one trap that will get you every time: your kitchen and pantry contents. If you don't have unhealthy foods in your home, then it's that much harder to eat the wrong things.

So, before you start your carb cycling journey, the first thing you should be doing is making sure you're well-stocked with the right foods – and getting rid of the wrong ones!

If you've been eating unhealthy convenience foods and snacks, you may need to purge before making a trip to the grocery store.

Go through all of your cabinets and storage areas, and find all the candy, chips, cookies, and commercially made, high salt crackers. If it's highly processed or salt, sugar, and fat laden, then it needs to go.

If the packages are already open, you can give them to family or friends (or take a homemade goodie basket to the office!). If you have any closed packages, you can always donate them to the local food bank or any local charitable organization. Most will be only too happy to take your closed and unused snack foods, and they'll still do some good!

Now that you've cleaned out your cupboards and got rid of all the high calorie, low nutrition snacks, there's room for stuff that's good for you. The good news is, good for you doesn't have to mean bland or tasteless! Here are some grocery shopping ideas to get you started:

Protein

- Lean red meat, poultry, and seafood
- Eggs (if you get Omega 3 enriched eggs, even better!)
- Dairy products, especially low-fat cottage cheese, plain yogurt, and similar products
- Beans, peas, and other legumes

Fats and Oils

- Olive oil
- Avocados
- Nuts and seeds (pumpkin seeds, sunflower seeds, etc.)
- Canola oil
- Oily fish

Fruits and Vegetables

- Sweet potatoes
- Tomatoes, cucumbers and other salad vegetables
- Various kinds of squash
- Onions
- Peppers
- Apples and pears
- Pineapples
- Berries, including strawberries, blueberries, etc.

Note: when choosing fruits, opt for fresh fruit rather than dried fruit, which are calorie dense but don't fill you up as much, and juice, which has very little nutritional value and a lot of sugar!

Grains

- Brown rice
- Quinoa
- Whole grain pasta
- Whole grain bread

- Bran
- Buckwheat noodles
- Wholegrain crackers (but check the salt and sugar content of commercial options!)

Note: Whenever possible, choose wholegrain grain products. The fiber in these products slows down digestion, which helps to prevent a spike in blood sugar.

Spices and Flavorings

One of the reasons we all hate "diet food" is that we always assume that it will be bland, boring, and basically inedible. That doesn't have to be the case. Even lower-calorie, healthier foods can be tasty if you use the right kind of flavorings. Stock your kitchen with a variety of:

- Hot sauce or sriracha
- Chili
- Garlic
- Ginger
- Lemon juice
- Herbs and spices
- Curry powders and pastes
- Soy sauce
- Honey

One of the best ways to make eating healthier more interesting and easier to stick to is to make it taste great. Various global cuisines can be adapted to healthy eating. It's much more fun to eat low carb honey garlic chicken or green curry than it is a boring salad!

General Shopping Tips

While your own carb cycling shopping trip will depend on the types of food you like to eat and the recipes you plan to try, you should always follow a few basic rules of thumb when you are shopping.

- Don't ever shop when you're hungry. You will always end up buying things that really aren't good for you.
- The more packaging a product has, the less likely it is to be good for you.
- Shop for the majority of your ingredients along the outside edges of the store. Middle aisles tend to have more processed items.
- Don't discount frozen, dried, or canned vegetables and beans (but avoid prepared canned foods!). They can have just as much nutritional value as their fresh counterparts, and they are much quicker to prepare!
- Make a list before you shop. You'll be less likely to buy things that aren't part of your plan.
- Audit your fridge, freezer, and pantry before you shop. It'll stop you from doubling up on items you already have enough of.
- If you struggle to avoid samples and sales on unhealthy items, take a shopping buddy with you. They'll help you to stay on the "straight and narrow."

Meal Prep

Another major factor in sticking to any diet is convenience. There's a reason why you find yourself in the drive-through with a large latte and a breakfast sandwich. We're all so busy every day that even when you have the best intentions, if you don't have food ready to go when you want it, you're going to struggle to stay on track.

Here are a few effortless ways to prep ahead of time, so you can grab something healthy and go:

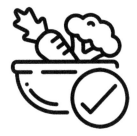

- Prepare overnight oats the night before. When you have to rush to get ready for work or school, it's much easier to eat a healthy breakfast!
- Bake your own egg and vegetable mini crustless quiches or "egg muffins" and individually wrap in wax paper to freeze. They can reheat in the microwave in a few minutes for an easy low carb breakfast.
- Make a variety of mason jar salads. Layer vegetables of your choice, add lean protein and an oil and vinegar-based dressing with herbs and spices for an easy lunch.
- Make extra-large batches of veggie chili, soup, or stir-fries. Portion them with brown rice (if applicable to the dish) and freeze individual servings. They're easy to pop in a lunch box for work or school, and they'll act as an ice pack to keep yogurt, fruits, or water cool.
- Create "snack packs" combining a few wholegrain crackers, apple slices and cheese, or peanut butter.
- Cut fruits and berries, and store portion-sized packs in the fridge. Add a plain yogurt, and you have a great snack or breakfast.
- Preboil eggs. A hard-boiled egg is a great high protein snack!
- Cut vegetables into sticks and store pre-portioned bags in

the fridge. A bag of veggie sticks with hummus, cottage cheese, or salsa is another great, easy snack.

Having snacks and meals ready to go when you're in a hurry will make you much more likely to stick to your diet.

Psyched and Ready

Hopefully, this chapter has demystified carb cycling, given you some idea of how it works, what you will be eating, and how to prepare for success.

Before you move on to the next parts of the book, which is all about getting started, take some time to make sure you're ready. Everything worth doing in life takes a little getting used to. The best way to ensure that you will succeed is to make sure you really want to do this, and you're fully committed to the process.

Changing your eating habits is the same as breaking any other habit. The best way to be sure it will work is to really want it. Not only will that set you up for success, but the more you do succeed, the more motivated you will be to continue.

On the flip side, if you're not really ready or committed, you're much more likely to slip and cheat, and the more you do that, the more you will make excuses why you can't keep going.

Make sure that the people in your life are on board too. If you have a family or a significant other, discuss how you will make your new eating plan work for them. The good news is that the meals you eat will still be healthy, and it's easy enough to add a few extra carbs to your partner's or children's meals. Trust me, most people won't be able to cope with making more than one meal every day, so you need to arrange this before you get started!

Carb cycling is not exactly easy. It's a lot easier to sustain than most highly restricted diets. However, you still need determination and discipline to make it work.

Now that we've got the science, information, and mindset covered, let's jump in and see how you get started.

ONE MUST EAT TO LIVE, NOT LIVE TO EAT.

Jean-Baptiste Poquelin

3

RECIPES

"When diet is wrong, medicine is of no use. When diet is correct, medicine is of no need". – *Ayurvedic Proverb*

While we wouldn't say that that is entirely accurate, there's no denying that maintaining a healthy weight and fitness level is the basis of good health. It also prepares you to be healthier overall. Even if you do fall ill, recovering tends to be easier if you're already in relatively good health.

A big part of that comes down to what we eat, but these days, many people either don't have time to cook or don't know where to start. We've got some great recipe ideas that are easy, use ingredients that you probably already have, and taste great. All the "ingredients" to help you stick to your new eating plan!

Note: Feel free to make some changes to the recipes. Does a recipe include something you simply can't stand? Switch it up for something you can! Allow yourself to get creative and stray a bit wherever you see fit.

If you have specific dietary restrictions or follow a diet (vegetarian or vegan as examples), you can easily modify the recipes to fit uniquely to you. Simply replace meats or items you may not be able to eat with your favorite alternatives such as tofu or extra vegetables. Add protein powder for an extra boost of protein.

Also, some recipes include sugar, syrup, or honey for taste. If you prefer to not have these, the recipes work great without them as well.

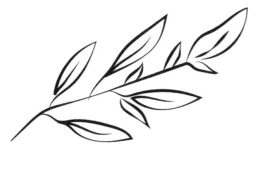

Breakfast

RECIPES

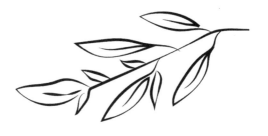

Ever heard the saying "breakfast is the most important meal of the day?" They weren't lying. Breakfast does precisely that – *breaks* your *fast*. Since carb cycling is all about regulating blood sugar, that's key.

Your body is programmed to try to regulate blood sugar levels. When you don't eat for a while, it starts signaling your cells to release stored glucose, keep it fueled, and, especially when you're sleeping, to prepare for the morning. This also interferes with insulin release and regulation.

When you wake up in the morning, your body is still doing this, and if you don't eat in the morning when you get up, your body will signal your liver to release even more glucose. Of course, we don't want that. We want our cells to use stored fat instead of carbs or glucose.

So, when it comes to eating in the morning, all the old wives were right!

We've collected some easy, tasty recipes that are both low and high carb, so you're ready for everything.

Low Carb

BREAKFAST

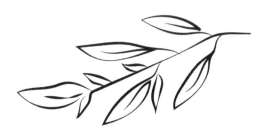

Breakfast is a tricky meal on low carb days. Think about your go-to options: toast, cereal, bagels. These recipes are tasty enough to take away the carb cravings, though, and still quick and easy to make.

EGG MUFFINS

Egg muffins are a perfect low carb snack. They're quick, can be made ahead, and frozen, and there are endless variations you can make to suit your mood and tastes. We've got three simple options for you to try.

INGREDIENTS:

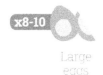
Large eggs
x8-10

Milk

Salt and pepper

Spinach and Feta

Frozen chopped spinach, defrosted

Crumbled feta

Tomato and Basil

Chopped tomato

Torn basil leaves

Chopped mozzarella

Tuna

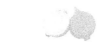
Chopped onions (sweated in a little olive oil until translucent)

Canned tuna

EGG MUFFINS

METHOD

1 Preheat oven to 350F.

2 Lightly grease a muffin pan with olive oil.

3 Whisk eggs with milk and season to taste

4 Mix your chosen add-ins together and place a generous tablespoon in the bottom of each muffin cup.

5 Fill each muffin cup to between 1/2 and 2/3 of the way full of egg mixture.

6 Gently stir and jiggle the tray to mix the the cups. You want the filling to be well distributed, but still in relatively large "chunks."

7 Bake for 10 minutes, or until the top of the muffins are lightly golden, and the egg is cooked through.

8 Remove from the oven, cool, and freeze for quick breakfast snacks.

BANANA NUT "PANCAKES"

Pancakes are a great breakfast choice, but they're not exactly "low carb." Except, they can be. This recipe uses no grain products at all and tastes great!

INGREDIENTS:

Ripe bananas, mashed

Large eggs, beaten

Oil for greasing pan

Tsp honey or maple syrup to serve

Peanut butter (optional)

Chopped peanuts (optional)

BANANA NUT "PANCAKES"

METHOD

1 Mix beaten eggs with bananas. Make sure the mixture is as smooth as possible.

2 Grease a heavy-based frying pan with oil and heat to medium on the stovetop.

3 Pour spoonsful of the banana mixture onto the pan and leave for a few minutes on each side. This mixture won't bubble like a typical pancake, so you will want to check by peeking under the edges from time to time.

4 Spread pancakes with peanut butter, if using, and drizzle with honey or a teaspoon of maple syrup.

5 Sprinkle with chopped nuts.

BAKED AVOCADOS

The combination of a creamy avocado, baked egg, and crispy bacon is the perfect way to start the day, and super simple to do! (One avocado serves two people.)

INGREDIENTS:

Avocado,
cut in half

Eggs

Salt and pepper
to taste

Rashers of bacon,
baked crispy
(if you bake the bacon
on a rack over a pan,
excess fat will drip out,
making this healthier!)

BAKED AVOCADOS
METHOD

1 Preheat oven to 350F.

2 Place avocado halves with the cut side facing up in a small oven-safe dish. Use balled up tinfoil if necessary, to stabilize each half.

3 Crack an egg into each half of the avocado, and season with salt and pepper.

4 Bake until the white of the egg is set, but the yolk is still runny and delicious.

5 Crumble bacon over avocado halves and serve.

SPICY SHAKSHUKA

Shakshuka is a spicy tomato-based egg dish that is super easy to make and great for breakfast! If you are cooking for a group, this is an excellent choice because it's easy to add crusty bread to their servings and leave it off your own.

INGREDIENTS:

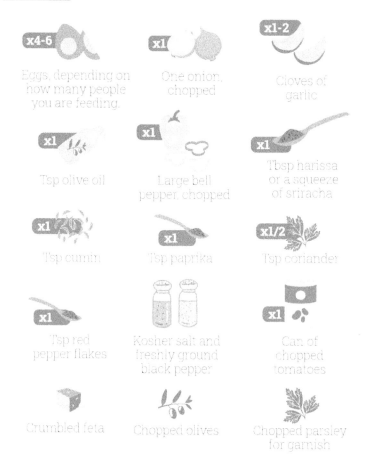

x4-6 Eggs, depending on how many people you are feeding.

x1 One onion, chopped

x1-2 Cloves of garlic

x1 Tsp olive oil

x1 Large bell pepper, chopped

x1 Tbsp harissa or a squeeze of sriracha

x1 Tsp cumin

x1 Tsp paprika

x1/2 Tsp coriander

x1 Tsp red pepper flakes

Kosher salt and freshly ground black pepper

x1 Can of chopped tomatoes

Crumbled feta

Chopped olives

Chopped parsley for garnish

SPICY SHAKSHUKA
METHOD

1 Preheat oven to 350F.

2 Heat a large oven-safe skillet and add oil.

3 Stir fry onions and garlic slowly over a low to medium heat, until they are translucent and fragrant.

4 Add bell pepper, spices, and seasoning to the pan, and continue stirring to release flavors.

5 Add the tomatoes to the pan and stir fry slowly, until some of the juice has evaporated.

6 Taste seasoning and adjust.

7 Using the back of a spoon, make hollows in the tomato mixture for the eggs, and crack one in each indentation.

8 Place the pan in the oven and bake until the egg whites are set.

9 Remove, top with feta, olives, and parsley and enjoy hot.

BREAKFAST FRITTATA

Eggs are a breakfast go-to for a very good reason.
This breakfast frittata has all the best parts of breakfast
in one easy to make, easy to love dish! Serves 2-3 people.
Add wholegrain toast for any diners who are not on a
low carb day!

INGREDIENTS:

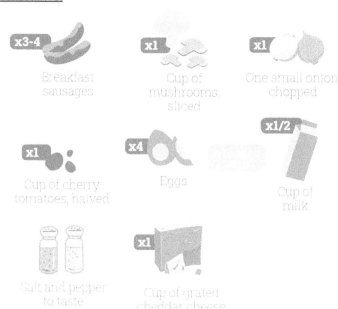

x3-4 Breakfast sausages

x1 Cup of mushrooms, sliced

x1 One small onion, chopped

x1 Cup of cherry tomatoes, halved

x4 Eggs

x1/2 Cup of milk

Salt and pepper to taste

x1 Cup of grated cheddar cheese

BREAKFAST FRITTATA

METHOD

1 Preheat oven to 350F.

2 Squeeze sausages out of their casings into a large oven-safe skillet.

3 Stir fry to brown, using a wooden spoon to break into small chunks.

4 When sausages are no longer pink, and some of the oil has rendered out of them, add the mushrooms and onions. Stir fry until onions have lost are translucent, and mushrooms have softened.

5 Add tomatoes to the pan, mix ingredients, and spread evenly over the bottom of the pan.

6 Pour seasoned egg and milk mixture into the pan and shake gently to ensure it covers the pan's base and surrounds all the ingredients.

7 Cook over low heat for a few minutes, until the bottom of the eggs are set.

8 Sprinkle cheese evenly over the top of the pan. Place pan in the oven and cook until the egg is set and the cheese has just started to bubble.

9 Serve wedges of the frittata.

BREAKFAST UN-SANDWICHES

Breakfast sandwiches are a fantastic easy to eat breakfast. Unfortunately, they're mostly bread, which makes them entirely unsuitable for low carb days. However, if you lose the bread and beef up the protein, you can have all the taste and convenience, without the carbs!

INGREDIENTS:

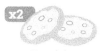
Breakfast sausage patties

Egg, whisked with a little milk and seasoned

Sliced avocado

Sliced tomato

BREAKFAST UN-SANDWICHES

METHOD

1 Add a little oil or oil spray to a frying pan and cook the sausage patties until they are cooked through and browned on both sides.

2 Grease a small non-stick pan and pour in the egg mixture. Cook gently on one side, flip, and cook the other.

3 Fold omelet to fit sausage patties.

4 Place one patty on a plate. Top with egg. Add avocado slices and tomato (both optional), season, and add condiments of your choice.

5 Top with another patty.

LOW CARB PUMPKIN SPICE MUESLI

Yes, cereal is one of your go-to breakfasts when you're in a hurry. Yes. It's usually full of carbs. But not this version! This muesli tastes like your go-to quick breakfast, but it's perfect for low carb days too! Make extra and store for a while but remember that some of the ingredients may spoil faster than your usual cereal, so eat as quickly as you can!

INGREDIENTS:

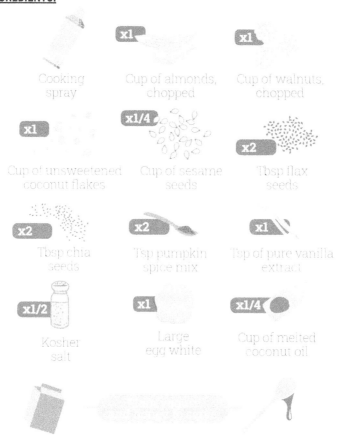

Cooking spray

x1 Cup of almonds, chopped

x1 Cup of walnuts, chopped

x1 Cup of unsweetened coconut flakes

x1/4 Cup of sesame seeds

x2 Tbsp flax seeds

x2 Tbsp chia seeds

x2 Tsp pumpkin spice mix

x1 Tsp of pure vanilla extract

x1/2 Kosher salt

x1 Large egg white

x1/4 Cup of melted coconut oil

LOW CARB PUMPKIN SPICE MUESLI

METHOD

1 Preheat oven to 350F.

2 Mix dry ingredients, including nuts, coconut flakes, and spices together.

3 Whisk egg white. Mix with coconut oil and toss with dry ingredient mix.

4 Spread onto a baking sheet and bake for about 20 minutes, or until golden brown and toasted. Watch carefully - they can burn quickly!

5 Allow the mix to cool, and then serve with plain yogurt, drizzled with honey.

Note: You can add additional nuts and seeds, like pumpkin seeds, sunflower seeds, and others, to this mix, or substitute your favorite ingredients as preferred.

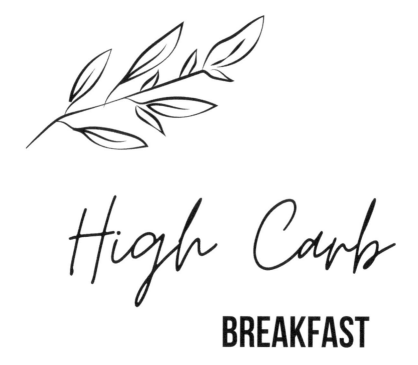

High Carb

BREAKFAST

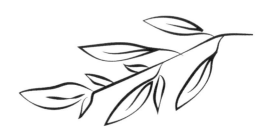

High carb breakfasts are a lot easier, because you can have cereal, muesli, or a make-ahead option like overnight oats. Most of these dishes are a little more decadent than that, but since it's a high carb day, you might as well make the most of it! Add a small serving of fresh fruit to any of these to boost the health factor.

STRAWBERRY CHEESECAKE FRENCH TOAST

French toast is a great breakfast, but when you add this cheesecake inspired filling, you take it to the next level! This breakfast tastes like a million bucks, but it's actually quick and easy to make. This is not an everyday breakfast dish, but if you're feeling like a bit of indulgence, it's a great way to start the day!

INGREDIENTS:

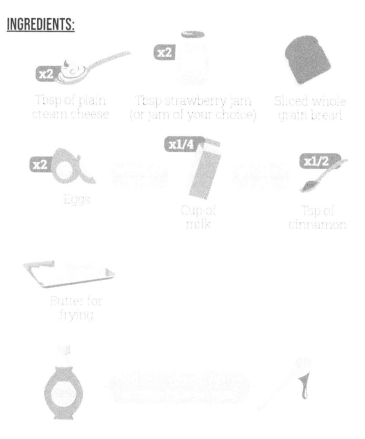

x2 Tbsp of plain cream cheese

x2 Tbsp strawberry jam (or jam of your choice)

Sliced whole grain bread

x2 Eggs

x1/4 Cup of milk

x1/2 Tsp of cinnamon

Butter for frying

STRAWBERRY CHEESECAKE FRENCH TOAST

METHOD

1 Melt butter in a skillet.

2 Mix cream cheese and jam to form a smooth paste.

3 Spread the cream cheese and jam mixture on bread and close to form a sandwich.

4 Dip each side of the sandwich in the egg mixture. Place the dipped sandwich in the buttered pan and cook slowly over a low to medium heat until golden. Flip and cook the other side.

5 Cut French toast sandwich in half diagonally, drizzle with honey or maple syrup and serve.

AVOCADO TOAST

Avocado toast has become a food legend over the past few years, and with good reason. It may sound like a simple dish, but it's the perfect base for many variations. Add crispy bacon and a soft fried egg, and you have an ideal handheld breakfast for high carb days!

INGREDIENTS:

Whole grain bread, lightly toasted and buttered

Small ripe avocado

Squeeze of lemon

Salt and pepper

Strips of bacon, baked or fried crispy

Egg, either fried or poached

Salsa

AVOCADO TOAST

METHOD

1 Mash the avocado with the lemon juice and salt and pepper.

2 Spoon avocado onto toast.

3 Top with crispy bacon.

4 Finish with egg and add salsa if using.

BREAKFAST HASH

Breakfast hash is a great one-pan breakfast option for days when you have a little more time. It is made with potatoes, which means it has a fair amount of carbs in it, but if you leave the skins on and add more vegetables, you can get a lot of good for you fiber.

INGREDIENTS:

 Large potato, cut into 1 cm cubes and parboiled until almost cooked and cooled

 Strips of bacon

 Small onion, chopped

 Green pepper, chopped

 Small, chopped tomato

 Salt and pepper to taste

 A soft fried egg to serve

BREAKFAST HASH

METHOD

1 Place bacon strips in a pan and cook over medium heat to render fat and become crispy. Remove from the pan and set aside to drain on a paper towel.

2 Add potatoes to the pan and cook until the edges are starting to brown.

3 Add chopped onion to the pan and fry gently until translucent.

4 Add green pepper and continue stir-frying. Onions should soften more, and potatoes should become golden brown.

5 Add chopped tomatoes to the pan and stir fry for about a minute to heat through.

6 Crumble bacon into the pan, season to taste, mix well, and turn onto a plate.

7 Top hash with egg and enjoy hot.

BLUEBERRY BREAKFAST STRATA

A strata is French toast's easier, more laid-back cousin.
You can make it the day before, leave it in the fridge,
and pop it in the oven when you wake up for a fuss-free
breakfast. Here's how you can make a blueberry version.
Substitute the berries for any other frozen fruit you like.
This dish serves a crowd, so it's great for a larger breakfast gathering!

INGREDIENTS:

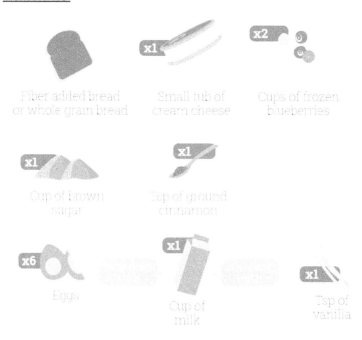

Fiber added bread
or whole grain bread

x1 Small tub of
cream cheese

x2 Cups of frozen
blueberries

x1 Cup of brown
sugar

x1 Tsp of ground
cinnamon

x6 Eggs

x1 Cup of
milk

x1 Tsp of
vanilla

BLUEBERRY BREAKFAST STRATA

METHOD

1 Grease a large, oven-proof dish.

2 Spread each slice of bread with cream cheese, and place in a single layer on the dish's bottom. You may need to cut slices to fit.

3 Sprinkle half the blueberries on the cream cheese layer.

4 Mix the brown sugar and cinnamon. Sprinkle 1/3 of the mixture over the blueberries.

5 Top with another layer of bread with cream cheese spread.

6 Sprinkle remaining berries over bread, along with 1/3 of the remaining sugar mixture.

7 Top with one more layer of bread, with the cream cheese spread facing down.

8 Pour the egg mixture evenly over the bread in the dish.

9 Sprinkle the top of the dish with the last of the sugar mixture.

10 When ready to bake, place in a 350F oven and bake for 40 to 50 minutes, or until egg custard is cooked and the top is golden brown.

11 Serve with plain yogurt and honey or maple syrup.

BREAKFAST BELT BAGEL

You've probably heard of the BLT, but when you add an egg, you get a BELT, and that's the perfect breakfast food! This version uses wholegrain bagels for added fiber, which makes for a slower release of carbs.

INGREDIENTS:

Wholegrain
bagel

Cream
cheese

Lettuce

Sliced
tomato

Crispy
bacon

Over easy
fried egg

BREAKFAST BELT BAGEL

METHOD

1 Slice bagel in half and toast lightly.

2 Spread both sides of the bagel with cream cheese.

3 Top with lettuce, tomato, and bacon.

4 Finish with a fried egg and serve.

WHOLEGRAIN TOAST WITH RICOTTA & BERRY COMPOTE

Toast is one of the most perfect breakfast foods ever invented. It's easy to make, and even if it's a high carb day, if you choose wholegrain toast, you're doing something good for your body. Add soft, creamy, delicious ricotta and sweet berries, and you've got a match made in breakfast heaven.

INGREDIENTS:

Wholegrain toast, buttered

Fresh ricotta cheese

Cups of frozen mixed berries

Cup of apple juice

Heaped teaspoon brown sugar

Toasted almonds

Honey to serve

WHOLEGRAIN TOAST WITH RICOTTA & BERRY COMPOTE

METHOD

1 Place berries, apple juice, and sugar in a small saucepan and let simmer slowly over medium heat until most of the liquid is evaporated.

2 Slightly mash the berries, leaving some larger chunks.

3 Crumble ricotta over toast and top with berry compote.

4 Top with a drizzle of honey and toasted almonds.

SCRAMBLED EGG & SMOKED SALMON BENEDICT

Eggs benedict are a brunch favorite. This version switches out fussy poached eggs for easy scrambled, adds delicious smoked salmon, and dresses them up with a dreamy hollandaise sauce. Use whole-wheat English muffins for added fiber.

INGREDIENTS:

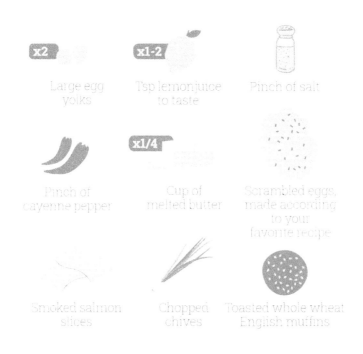

x2 Large egg yolks

x1-2 Tsp lemon juice to taste

Pinch of salt

Pinch of cayenne pepper

x1/4 Cup of melted butter

Scrambled eggs, made according to your favorite recipe

Smoked salmon slices

Chopped chives

Toasted whole wheat English muffins

SCRAMBLED EGG & SMOKED SALMON BENEDICT

METHOD

1 Mix the first five ingredients well in a microwave-safe glass jug.

2 Microwave on high for 15-20 seconds.

3 Use an immersion blender to blend into a smooth and creamy sauce.

4 Top toasted muffins with scrambled eggs and smoked salmon. Drizzle with easy hollandaise, and top with chopped chives.

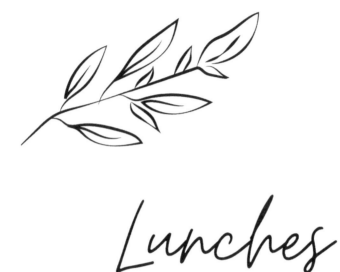

Lunches

& DINNERS

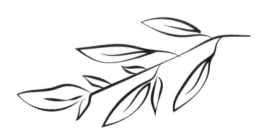

Lunch and dinner are a little easier to adapt to carb cycling because we're not as used to reaching for baked goods as we are in the morning! These dishes are quick, easy, and tasty. They are also proof that you can still eat delicious, flavorful meals even when you're watching carbs.

Low Carb

LUNCHES & DINNERS

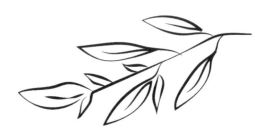

The key to staying full when you're on a low carb day is to add a little more protein and fat to your meals. Add fruit and vegetables, and you can still have a delicious meal that tastes great but won't spike your blood sugar!

SPAGHETTI SQUASH & MEATBALLS

You don't have to skip Italian night just because it's a low carb day. Just switch the pasta for garlic butter spaghetti squash.

INGREDIENTS:

Small spaghetti squash, cut in half and with seeds scooped out

Butter

Mixed herbs

Parmesan cheese

Small pack of lean ground beef

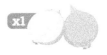

Small onion finely chopped or minced

Cloves garlic crushed or grated

Egg

Barbecue or Italian seasoning, to taste

Salt and pepper to taste

Jarred or home-made marinara sauce to serve

Grated parmesan to serve

SPAGHETTI SQUASH & MEATBALLS

METHOD

1 Preheat oven to 350F.

2 Grease a baking sheet. Place squash cut side down on the sheet and place in the oven.

3 Roast for about 30 minutes, or until a knife inserted in the squash slides in easily.

4 While squash is roasting, combine beef, finely chopped onion, garlic, egg, and seasoning. Mix well to combine, and using wet hands, form into small balls. Place balls in a greased oven-proof dish.

5 When squash is cooked through, remove from the oven and set aside to cool.

6 Place meatballs in the oven and cook for about 20 - 30 minutes, or until browned and cooked through. Smaller meatballs will cook faster.

7 Heat marinara in a pot and add meatballs. Heat through.

8 Scrape flesh from cooled squash into a bowl.

9 Mix in butter, herbs, and cheese.

10 Place squash on plates, top with meatballs and sauce, and sprinkle with cheese.

CAJUN CHICKEN SALAD

Main course salads are an excellent choice for low carb lunches and dinners. They're easy to make, taste great, and don't leave you feeling deprived. This Cajun version is spicy and delicious!

INGREDIENTS:

 Boneless, skinless chicken breasts

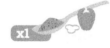 Tbsp paprika

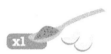 Tbsp garlic powder

 Tsp dried oregano

 Tsp dried thyme

 Tsp salt

  Black pepper and cayenne pepper to taste

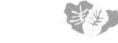 Lettuce

 Tomatoes

Cucumbers

 Thinly sliced red onions

 Sliced avocados

 Cup full-fat yogurt

Cup full-fat mayonnaise

 Squeeze of lime

 Tsp of spice mixture (reserved from mix made above)

CAJUN CHICKEN SALAD

METHOD

1 Mix all spices together until fully incorporated.

2 Remove chicken tenders, and lightly pound chicken to flatten slightly.

3 Sprinkle both sides of chicken breast fillets and tenders liberally with the spice mix.

4 Heat a tbsp of olive oil in a skillet.

5 Cook chicken over a medium-high heat until fully cooked through. If the pan dries out, add a little water to loosen the spice mix and prevent burning.

6 When chicken is cooked through, and the spice mix/panjuices have created a dark, spicy crust, remove chicken from the heat and set aside to cool slightly.

7 Build salad using lettuce, tomatoes, cucumber, and onions, finish with avocado.

8 Mix mayonnaise and yogurt together and add spice mix and lime.

9 Slice chicken and place on top of the salad, then drizzle with dressing.

POACHED SOLE WITH LEMON CAPER SAUCE & ROASTED BROCCOLI

Sole is a very light fish with a very mild flavor. A lemon, butter, and caper sauce takes it to the next level, and serving it with roasted broccoli is a great easy, light weeknight dinner.

INGREDIENTS:

Sole fillets

Cup of butter

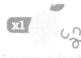
Lemon, juiced and zested

Tsp capers

Mixed herbs

Salt and pepper

Bag of frozen broccoli

Tbsp olive oil

POACHED SOLE WITH LEMON CAPER SAUCE & ROASTED BROCCOLI

METHOD

1 Preheat oven to 350F.

2 Place sole in a deep-frying pan, add enough water to just barely cover, season, and poach until the fish is just cooked and opaque.

3 Carefully remove the fish to an oven dish and set aside.

4 Empty pan, then melt butter and add lemon juice, zest, seasoning, and herbs. Cook over medium heat until the butter is just starting to brown a little.

5 Pour over the fish and keep warm.

6 Toss broccoli with olive oil and seasoning.

7 Arrange in a single layer on a baking sheet, and bake for 20 to 30 minutes, or until fully heated and cooked through and beginning to brown on the edges.

8 Serve fish with sauce and broccoli on the side.

CAULIFLOWER "MAC" & CHEESE WITH BACON

Mac and cheese is the ultimate comfort food. But it's not exactly low carb. This cauliflower version has all the cheesy goodness and very little of the carbs!

INGREDIENTS:

Head of cauliflower cut into florets and steamed until soft.

Cup of milk

Tbsp butter

Tsp cornstarch dissolved in a little more milk

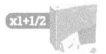
Cups of strong cheddar

cup of additional cheddar

Salt and pepper to taste

Strips of crispy bacon, crumbled

CAULIFLOWER "MAC" & CHEESE WITH BACON

METHOD

1 Preheat oven to 350F.

2 Arrange cauliflower in an oven-proof dish. Heat milk in a small saucepan, add butter, and melt. Season to taste.

3 When milk is almost at boiling point, pour cornstarch slurry into the milk, and continue heating, stirring to prevent lumps from forming.

4 Continue stirring until the milk mixture begins to thicken.

5 When the desired thickness has been reached, add cheese to the sauce mixture. Stir until melted. Pour cheese sauce over the cauliflower, covering completely.

6 Sprinkle additional cheese and chopped bacon over the cheese sauce.

7 Bake in the oven until the top of the cheese is melting and bubbling.

STEAK, ROASTED TOMATOES, AND CAULIFLOWER "MASHED"

Meat and potatoes, without the potatoes, but with all the taste! It's the perfect fancy dinner that's still easy to make and tastes great! This dish works best if you have a cast-iron pan, but a heavy stainless steel one will work as well. Avoid non-stick because they don't get hot enough to properly sear the steak.

INGREDIENTS:

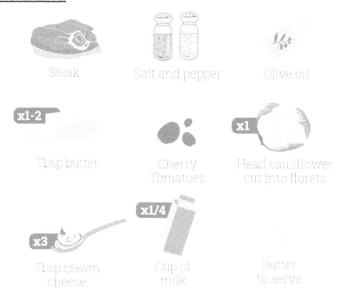

Steak

Salt and pepper

Olive oil

x1-2
Tbsp butter

Cherry Tomatoes

x1
Head cauliflower cut into florets

x3
Tbsp cream cheese

x1/4
Cup of milk

Butter to serve

STEAK, ROASTED TOMATOES, AND CAULIFLOWER "MASHED"

METHOD

1 Preheat oven to 350F.

2 Heat a cast-iron skillet until very hot.

3 Lightly oil steak and season both sides with salt and pepper.

4 Place steak in the hot pan, leaving to sear entirely before turning to repeat on the other side.

5 Turn off heat and add butter to the pan.

6 Add cherry tomatoes to the pan and coat with butter and pan juices.

7 Place pan in the oven to finish.

8 Boil cauliflower in a little water until soft.

9 Drain and mash with cream cheese, milk, and seasoning.

10 When steak and tomatoes are cooked, serve with cauliflower mash, topped with butter.

CAULIFLOWER "FRIED RICE"

This recipe is super quick and tastes like Chinese takeout, but without the carbs.

INGREDIENTS:

Vegetable oil for frying (or a mixture of olive and sesame oil)

 Eggs, beaten

 Salt

 x3-4 Chopped green onions

 x2 Minced garlic cloves

 x1 Tsp grated ginger

 x4 Tbsp soy sauce

 x1 Tsp brown sugar

 Pinch of chili flakes

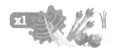 x1 Cup of frozen mixed vegetables

 x1 Tsp rice vinegar

 x1 Head of cauliflower, grated

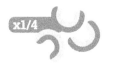 x1/4 Cup of cashews, chopped

 x1/2 Cup cooked ham or chicken, diced (optional)

CAULIFLOWER "FRIED RICE"

METHOD

1 Heat oil in a wok or large frying pan.

2 Add green onions, spices, soy sauce, and sugar.

3 Stir for a moment until fragrant.

4 Add eggs and quickly stir fry to scramble.

5 Add frozen vegetables and cauliflower to the pan and stir fry for 3 - 4 minutes. Add a drizzle of water if the pan is too dry.

6 When the vegetables are cooked, add cashews and chicken or ham, and stir to heat through.

7 Serve with more soy sauce for seasoning to taste if desired.

VEGETARIAN CHILLI

Carb free doesn't have to be meat-heavy. You can make tasty meals without carbs or meat. Here's a great one!

INGREDIENTS:

Tbsp oil
for frying

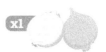
Medium onion,
chopped

Cloves garlic,
chopped

Small green pepper,
seeded and cut
into chunks

Large can of
red kidney beans,
drained and rinsed

Can of
chopped
tomatoes

Sachet of
chili seasoning

Salt and pepper
to taste

Cups of
vegetable stock

Plain yogurt, cheese,
and hot sauce to serve

VEGETARIAN
CHILLI

1 Heat oil in a large, heavy-based saucepan.

2 Fry onion with a little salt until translucent and just starting to brown.

3 Add green pepper and stir fry for about a minute.

4 Stir in seasoning sachet, salt and pepper, and cook until fragrant.

5 Add beans, tomatoes, and vegetable stock. Cook over medium heat until vegetables are softened and soup has thickened - about 40 minutes.

6 Serve chili with a swirl of plain yogurt and grated cheese.

7 Add hot sauce to taste.

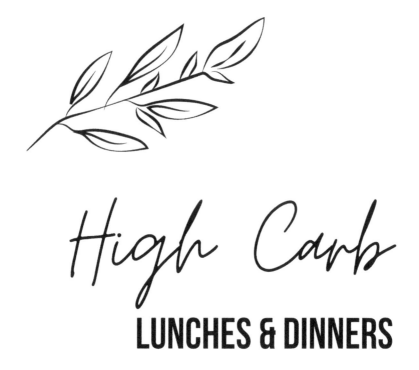

High Carb

LUNCHES & DINNERS

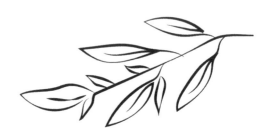

High carb days are a lot more forgiving in terms of lunches and dinners. However, you should still opt for higher fiber, less processed carbs, just to keep your blood sugar stable and to avoid overly processed foods. Whether you're carb cycling or not, processed foods are never a great choice.

WHOLE GRAIN PITA "PIZZAS"

Whole grain pitas make fantastic personal pizzas, and since everyone has their own, you can choose whatever you like to top yours with! Choose wholegrain pitas, so you get a little more fiber with your meal.

INGREDIENTS:

Whole grain
pitas

Commercial
pizza sauce

Chopped ham
or chicken,
pepperoni, ground
beef, or other meats
of your choice

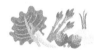
Chopped vegetables,
such as mushrooms,
peppers, onions,
or tomatoes

Avocado,
pineapple,
or anchovies

Grated
mozzarella

Grated cheddar
cheese

WHOLE GRAIN PITA "PIZZAS"

METHOD

1 Preheat oven to 350F.

2 Spread a thin layer of pizza sauce over each pita pizza. Don't use too much, or you will have a soggy crust and toppings that slide off.

3 Top with meats and cheeses of your choice.

4 Sprinkle liberally with cheese.

5 Bake until cheese is melted and bubbling.

6 Remove and allow to cool for a few minutes before slicing.

GREEK LAMB KEBABS, COUSCOUS, AND TZATZIKI

Greek lamb kebabs are made from ground lamb, but if you have trouble finding some or prefer beef, you can cheat and use that instead! This dish is quick and easy to make but looks like you spent a lot of time on it, so it's great for entertaining!

INGREDIENTS:

Cloves of garlic, crushed

Tsp salt

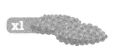
Pound of ground lamb (or beef)

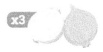
Tbsp grated onion

Tbsp chopped parsley

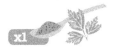
Tbsp ground coriander

Tsp ground cumin

Tsp cayenne pepper

Ground black pepper

Juice of one lemon

Cucumber, grated

Cup of thick Greek yogurt

Lemon juice

Clove crushed garlic

Chopped mint

Crumbled feta cheese

Couscous, prepared according to directions, using chicken stock instead of water

Chopped tomato

Chopped cucumber

Salt and pepper

Lemon zest

Mixed herbs

Canned chickpeas, drained and rinsed

GREEK LAMB KEBABS, COUSCOUS, AND TZATZIKI

METHOD

1 Preheat oven to 350F.

2 Mix all of the first batch of ingredients together well.

3 Form meat mixture into slightly elongated meatballs on bamboo or wooden skewers. Place on a lightly greased baking sheet and place in the oven to cook.

4 Squeeze the grated cucumber to remove excess water. Mix with remaining tzatziki ingredients. Mix all couscous salad ingredients together.

5 When kebabs are cooked, serve on a bed of couscous salad with tzatziki.

BETTER TEX MEX BURGERS & FRIES

Burgers aren't usually what you think of when you think of healthy eating, but you can make them a better choice with a few tweaks. This version uses opts for grilled patties and sweet potato fries.

INGREDIENTS:

High quality frozen or home bade beef burgers

Wholegrain buns

Mashed avocado

Jarred salsa

Sliced Cheese

Lettuce

Tomato

Frozen sweet potato oven fries

BETTER TEX MEX BURGERS & FRIES

METHOD

1 Cook sweet potato fries according to the manufacturer's directions.

2 Cook burgers on a lightly greased grill or griddle pan.

3 Slice buns and "butter" with mashed avocado. Top with lettuce and tomato slices.

4 When burgers are cooked, place on bun and immediately top with cheese, so that cheese melts.

5 Finish with salsa and add more on the side for dipping fries.

6 Season fries and serve.

LOADED BAKED POTATOES

Potatoes have a lot of starch in them, but they're also full of a lot of good things. Baked potatoes with their skins on are also full of fiber, which is always a good thing. Microwaved baked potatoes are very quick and easy to make too!

INGREDIENTS:

Medium potatoes, scrubbed

Chopped spring onions

Diced tomatoes

Chopped crispy bacon

Plain yogurt

Cheddar cheese

LOADED BAKED POTATOES

METHOD

1 Poke holes in potatoes with a fork, place on a plate, and microwave for about 2 minutes for each medium-sized potato you are cooking. Check every few minutes to see if the potatoes are soft.

2 When they are cooked, a knife should pierce them easily.

3 Allow potatoes to cool slightly, then cut a cross in the top and squeeze to open.

4 Using a teaspoon, spoon yogurt into the potato, mash into the flesh slightly to mix and add a little more to the top.

5 Top with diced tomatoes, spring onions, and bacon. Sprinkle potatoes with cheddar cheese, and then place under the grill in the oven until the cheese is melted and bubbling.

Note: Baked potatoes can be topped with several different toppings, from spicy beans to tuna salad and more. Topping with cheese and grilling takes them to the next level!

JAPANESE STYLE SALMON BOWLS

Lightly battered salmon, crispy vegetables, brown rice, and sesame sauce. It's the perfect way to eat carbs while still sticking to a healthy eating plan!

INGREDIENTS:

Salmon fillets

Seasoned flour for dusting

Oil for frying

Finely grated carrots

Bean sprouts

Thinly sliced cucumber

Japanese style sesame dressing

Cooked brown rice to serve

JAPANESE STYLE SALMON BOWLS

1 Lightly dust salmon fillets in seasoned flour.

2 Heat oil in a frying pan.

3 Fry salmon over medium heat, taking care not to burn flour coating, until cooked through.

4 Flash fry carrots and bean sprouts.

5 Spoon brown rice into bowl.

6 Top with grated carrots, bean sprouts, and cucumber slices.

7 Finish with salmon, and drizzle with Japanese style sesame sauce.

TUNA FISH CAKES WITH SALAD

Canned tuna might not be the first thing you think of when you hear healthier eating, but it's actually a low fat, high protein choice that's easy and cheap to keep on hand. These fish cakes transform it from mediocre to amazing!

INGREDIENTS:

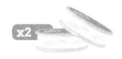

x2

Cans
of tuna

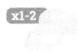

x1-2

2 small or one large
potato, peeled, cooked
and mashed, and cooled

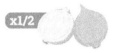

x1/2

Onion,
finely chopped

Mixed herbs

Lemon zest

x1

Large egg,
beaten

Flour
to dredge

Lemon weges
to serve

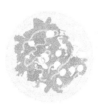

Garden salad to serve

TUNA FISH CAKES WITH SALAD

METHOD

1 Mix tuna, cooled mashed potato, onion, herbs, lemon zest, and egg. The mixture should be well combined but still have a few larger chunks of fish.

2 Chill the mixture. It is much easier to shape into cakes if cold!

3 When cold, form heaped tablespoons of mixture into patties. Dredge in flour, and place in a frying pan with about ¼ inch hot oil to shallow fry.

4 Fry over medium heat until golden on one side, then flip to cook the other side too.

5 Drain cooked fishcakes on kitchen paper, and then serve accompanied by lemon and salad.

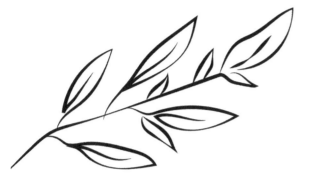

Snacks

As much as we would like to eat carefully balanced, home-cooked meals every time we're hungry, the truth is that sometimes you just need something quick on the go. These quick and easy snacks are a great choice when you're short on time!

Low Carb Snacks

Low carb snacks are easier than you think. Here are some good ideas:

- Hard-boiled eggs. You can precook some and keep them in the fridge for a few days.
- Half an avocado with lemon, salt, and pepper.
- Mixed nuts.
- A slice or wedge of cheese.
- Cream cheese with celery sticks or crudité.
- Plain yogurt with fresh berries. Berries are actually much lower in carbs than most fruit.

Healthy High Carb Snacks

Just because you can eat carbs today doesn't mean you should be reaching for the chips. Here are some healthier alternatives:

- Whole grain crackers with cheese or peanut butter.
- Fruit that isn't berries, like apples or peaches. Add a little protein and fat, like a slice of cheese or a handful of nuts, to balance it out.
- Rice cakes with cream cheese.

Whether you are on a carb cycling diet or not, it's a good idea to eat every two to three hours, so your blood sugar stays relatively stable. That means you should be aiming to eat about five or six times a day. Three meals, and two or three snacks in between.

11

SAMPLE CARB CYCLING PLANS

Now that you know what you can eat, and how you might go about preparing for the various days of your carb cycling plan, we've put together a sample carb cycling plan that you might use to get started.

Low Carb / High Carb Plan

In this example, we've combined some of the recipes in this book into a simple low carb day, high carb day cycle.

SAMPLE LOW-CARB/HIGH-CARB PLAN

	BREAKFAST	LUNCH	DINNER
MON	Egg Muffins	Cajun Chicken Salad	Spaghetti Squash & Meatballs
TUES	Avocado Toast	Whole Grain Pita Pizzas	Tuna Fish Cakes With Salad
WED	Banana Nut Pancakes	Cauliflower Fried Rice	Baked Teriyaki Salad & Vegetables
THURS	Breakfast Hash	Grilled Cheese & Tomato Soup	Greek Lamb Kebabs w/ couscous
FRI	Baked Avocado	Grilled Steak Salad	Vegetarian Chili
SAT	Breakfast BELT Bagel	Loaded Baked Potato	Burgers & Sweet Potato Fries
SUN	Spicy Shakshuka	Vegetarian Chili	Japanese Style Salmon Bowls

Low Carb, Medium Carb, High Carb Plan

You might find that having your plan built around three days (one low, one medium, and one high) works better for you. This plan is based on that scenario.

SAMPLE LOW-CARB/MEDIUM-CARB/ HIGH-CARB PLAN

	BREAKFAST	LUNCH	DINNER
MON	Banana Nut Pancakes	Baked Avocados	Spaghetti Squash & Meatballs
TUES	Breakfast Frittata	Cauliflower Mac & Cheese	Tuna Fish Cakes With Salad
WED	Strawberry Cheesecake French Toast	Whole Grain Pita Pizzas	Loaded Baked Potatoes
THURS	Breakfast Un-Sandwiches	Vegetarian Chili	Poached Sole w/ Lemon, Capers, & Broccoli
FRI	Low-Carb Pumpkin Spice Muesli	Cajun Chicken Salad	Greek Lamb Kebabs, Tzatziki, & Couscous Salad
SAT	Toast with Ricotta & Berry Compote	Quesadilla & Salsa	Chicken Alfredo
SUN	Egg Muffins	Cauliflower Fried Rice	Vegetarian Chili

As you can see, carb cycling does not mean eating nothing but limp lettuce. It's not boring, and because you alternate high and low carb days, you won't ever be craving carbs so badly that you fall completely off the wagon.

Now that we've covered the food part of the equation, we need to look at the rest of the plan: exercise.

THE DOCTOR OF THE
FUTURE WILL NO
LONGER TREAT THE
HUMAN FRAME WITH
DRUGS, BUT RATHER
WILL CURE AND
PREVENT DISEASE
WITH NUTRITION.

Thomas Edison

12

EXERCISE

You might have already noticed that as far as diet and lifestyle plans go, carb cycling is a reasonably moderate, balanced concept. While exercise is a crucial part of the plan, it follows the same formula, which means that you'll never have to work yourself to a standstill every day of the week.

Some days you will work harder and sweat more, and others will be more laid back and focus more on things like light strength training, flexibility, or just hitting a step goal.

Unfortunately, even if you were to be a "couch tomato" and sit on the couch without moving, only eating salads, you wouldn't be what most people would consider healthy. As soon as you changed your diet, even a little, you'd gain weight rapidly.

The older you get, the lower your basal metabolic rate will drop, too, so even if you used to be able to get away with it, it will eventually catch up to you.

Choosing a moderate, balanced diet and exercise plan like carb cycling is the best choice, no matter what stage of life you're in. Still, the sooner you get used to a lifestyle like this, the better it will be in the long term.

High Carbs, High Energy!

Remember that equation, where the more calories you eat, the more you need to work out to lose weight and keep it off? The same applies to carb cycling, except in this case, it's carbs, not calories.

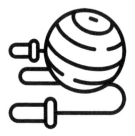

On the days when you eat a lot of carbs, you need to work harder to burn them off, so when you have a low-calorie day, your body starts burning fat.

That means that high carb days are the days you're probably going to sweat!

Some examples of good high carb day workouts are:

- Power walking or jogging
- Cycling
- Swimming
- High energy sports like tennis
- Cardio circuits or spin classes at the gym
- Aerobics or tae-bo style workouts
- HIIT
- Intense strength training

The amount of exercise you will need to do on any high carb day will vary based on your individual diet plan, but in most cases, you will need to do about half an hour of your chosen activity to burn enough carbs off.

Low Carbs, Lower Energy

The best thing about the carb cycling plan is that you always get a "day off" after doing the hard work. So, you watch what you eat and work out hard one day, and the next day you can have the bagel and take it a little easier with the sweating.

On low carb days, you don't have to do as much to burn off carbs. Since you should be eating the right kinds of foods and sticking to your daily calorie limit regardless of whether it's a high or low carb day, you should still lose weight.

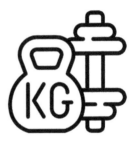

Some examples of the type of activities you could do on low energy days might be:

- Yoga or Pilates
- Walking or hiking at a slower pace
- Low-intensity weight and strength training

Your workouts on low carb days don't have to be as intense, but you should still aim for about half an hour of conscious activity on those days. Make sure you're moving, even if it's just a walk around a park at lunchtime or a playful activity with your kids after work.

Exercise Not Optional

There are some diets out there that promise that if you restrict your calories to half what they should be or eat something bland and boring for a week, the pounds will melt right off and stay gone, but that's just not true.

Carb cycling is not one of those diets. In fact, it's more of a lifestyle plan than a diet at all.

You won't have to run yourself ragged in the gym every moment, but you're going to have to do some work to get the results you want.

If you're dreading getting off the couch and committing to some sort of physical activity every day, though, there is a silver lining.

That is, the more you work out, the fitter you will get, and the easier it will become. You might even learn to like it.

The other crucial fact is that muscle will always burn more energy than fat. So even if you might not lose weight as quickly when you eat right and exercise right, you will lose inches faster, and you'll actually keep losing them faster because you'll be building more muscle every time you get moving.

Your basal metabolic rate will rise, and your body, instead of being a sneak and hiding new deposits of fat in every spare place it can find, will actually become your fat-burning ally.

Sample Full-Body Workout

This book is meant to help you get started with carb cycling and is not specifically an exercise guide. Still, we wanted you to have a simple workout option in case you needed help getting started and some motivation. So we created a simple full-body workout to help you get moving and become a healthier you! This workout doesn't require you to have any equipment and can be done from pretty much anywhere. It also combines some high-intensity exercises to quickly burn calories along with some lower intensity exercises that will still have you feeling the burn. We have placed some recommended numbers for the amount of repetitions and sets to perform for each activity. If you enjoy other workouts and exercises, make sure to follow those. It will be more likely for you to continue doing them and making progress. If you are just getting started, however, give these a try.

Start slowly, and if you notice that the number of repetitions is unrealistic for you, change the amount to something more suitable. You will see improvements week by week. If, on the other hand, the number of repetitions is too low, increase your workload. Try to perform each exercise until the last 2-3 repetitions are challenging.

Now, before we get started, it is crucial to consult with a medical professional to make sure you are fit for any strenuous activity. Since the workout is based on your body weight, it may be intensive on certain joints like your knees and elbows. If you feel uncomfortable or in pain throughout any exercise, stop the training right away. Injuring yourself unnecessarily will not bring you any closer to achieving your goals. Stay safe as you continue to push your progress forward.

Let's get started!

Start your full-body workout with a warm-up circuit. Complete 3 sets of high knees, jumping jacks, and lateral toe taps as shown in the diagrams, to get your blood pumping and your body ready to work. Complete each exercise for 30 seconds before moving on to the next one. Take a 30 second break in between each set.

HIGH KNEES

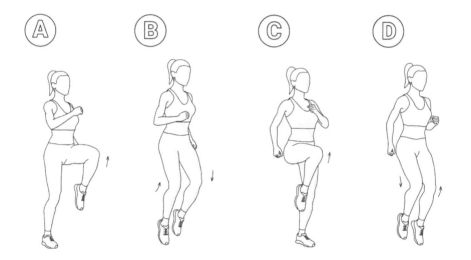

JUMPING JACKS

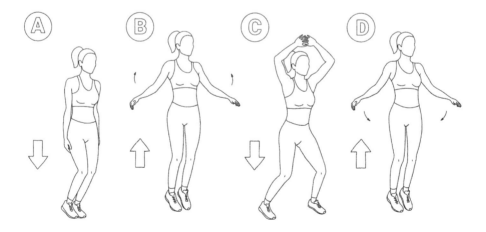

LATERAL TOE TAPS

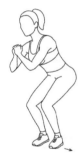

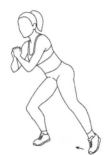

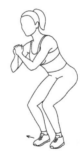

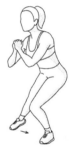

SQUATS

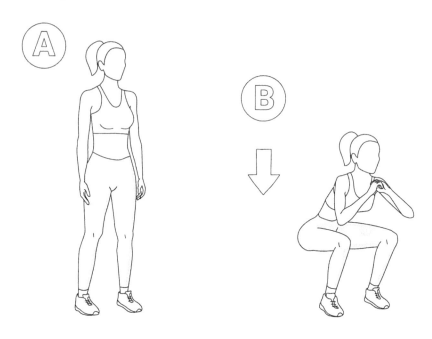

Complete an air squat by standing straight with your feet facing forward shoulder-width apart. Squat by moving your hips down and back. Aim to keep your back straight rather than curved forward and keep your heels flat on the floor. Try to get your hips lower than your knees. Don't worry if you do not yet have this range of motion. Keep at it, and over time, you will be able to get lower into your squat. Aim to complete 3 sets of 12 to 15 repetitions.

JUMP SQUATS

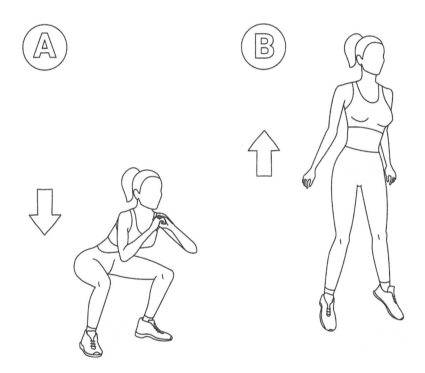

Complete a jump squat by lowering yourself into a squat and exploding up into a jump. As soon as you land, continue by lowering yourself into a squat again and repeat the process. Aim to complete 3 sets of 8 repetitions.

PUSH-UP

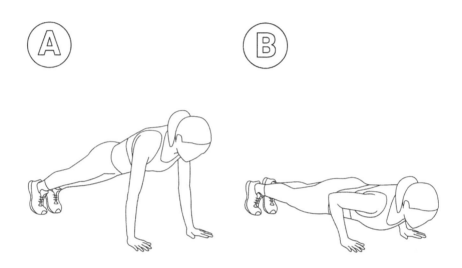

Complete a push up by getting down on all fours and placing your hands slightly wider than your shoulders. Straighten your arms and legs into a plank position and lower your body by bending your elbows. Keep your core flexed, so you do not bend at your hips. Lower your body until your chest nearly touches the floor, then push yourself back up into the starting plank position. Aim to complete 3 sets of 10 repetitions.

Note: if you can complete more, continue until your last 3 repetitions are difficult.

BURPEE

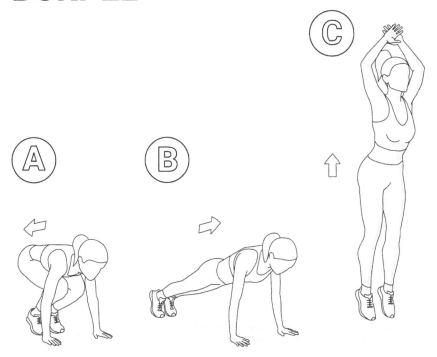

You will definitely develop a love-hate relationship with this one but a burpee is a great exercise to quickly train pretty much every muscle in your body. Start in a neutral position with your feet shoulder-width apart and your arms at your sides. Lower your body into a low squat and lower your arms to the floor as you transfer your weight forward, quickly moving into plank position. Jump your feet back towards your hands and reach your arms over your head as you jump up into the air. After you land, immediately lower back into a squat for your next repetition. Aim for 3 sets of 10-15 repetitions.

Note: this is a strenuous exercise, make sure to listen to your body and don't overexert yourself.

TRICEPS DIPS

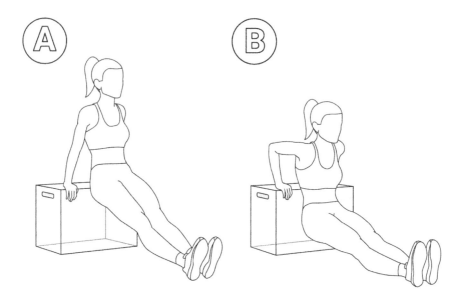

Find a stable surface (chair, step, bench, etc.) and sit on it. Grip the edge next to your hips and with your legs extended, press into your palms and lift your body up. Slide forward slightly and lower yourself until your elbows are bent around 90 degrees. Slowly push yourself up to your starting position and repeat. Aim to complete 3 sets of 10 repetitions.

PIKE PUSH-UPS

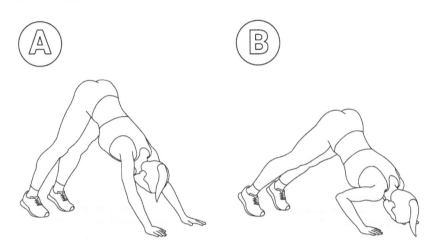

Complete a pike push up by getting down on all fours and placing your hands slightly wider than your shoulders. Straighten your arms and lift up your hips so that your body forms an upside-down V. Try to keep your arms and legs as straight as possible. Bend your elbows as if you were doing a regular push up and lower your body until your head nearly touches the floor. Push yourself back up to your starting position and repeat. Aim to complete 3 sets of 5-8 repetitions.

MOUNTAIN CLIMBERS

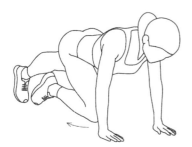

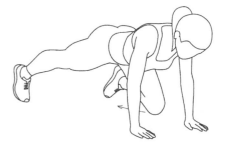

Complete mountain climbers, by getting on your hands and knees and then in a plank position. While balancing your weight evenly, lift your right knee, and bring it towards your right hand. Hold this position for half a second, and then in a smooth motion, switch your legs while keeping your arms in the same place. Aim to complete 3 sets of 20-30 seconds of this exercise.

SEATED CRUNCH

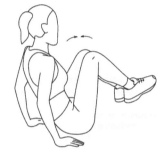 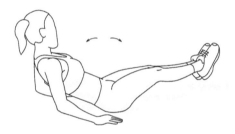

To complete a seated crunch, start in a seated position and place your hands to your sides slightly behind your hips. Lean back slightly and lift your knees, as shown in the diagram. Lean back further as you extend your legs away. After stretching out your legs, contract them back to your starting position and repeat. Aim to complete 3 sets of 10-15 repetitions.

FULL
PLANK

LOW
PLANK

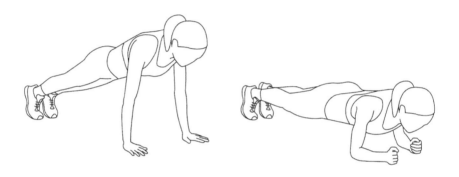

This is a great exercise to keep your back healthy and to strengthen your core. Complete a plank by getting into one of the two plank positions shown in the diagram above. Aim to complete 3 sets of 20-30 seconds.

LOVE YOURSELF ENOUGH TO LIVE A HEALTHY LIFESTYLE.

Jules Robson

MAINTENANCE

Have you ever wondered, when you finish that three week long "diet," what you're supposed to do next?

If you just go back to your old habits, you'll just gain all the weight back, with interest.

In fact, research shows that 80 to 95% of people who lose 10% or more of their body weight will gain it back, and more.

Why?

Because when we're on a "diet," we believe there's an end date. The day you reach your goal weight. Or the day you can fit into the pants you wore in high school. As soon as you reach that date, you're finished with your weight loss journey, and you can go back to normal.

The problem with that is if you've been on a ridiculous diet that requires you to eat foods you can't pronounce, or so little of anything that you're constantly fainting like a Victorian lady, you can't keep it up. But you haven't learned any other healthy way of keeping the weight off, so normal means the same old bad habits.

Before you know it, you're heading in the wrong direction, with no clue what to do except stop eating anything vaguely tasty for weeks or months.

It's a vicious cycle, and it needs to be broken.

Fortunately, a maintenance system is built right into the carb cycling lifestyle plan, and it's easy to adapt when you reach your goal weight.

Weaning Yourself Off Carb Cycling

If you're doing carb cycling right, you're going to see a slow, gradual, reliable weight loss. This is not a crash diet where you can quickly lose a lot of weight and then gain it back again almost overnight. But that also means that your new eating plan will start to become a habit, and we all know habits can be hard to break.

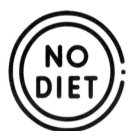 Even if you are mentally prepared to end your "diet," your body won't like a sudden change, so when you reach your goal weight, it's essential to spend some time weaning yourself off your eating plan.

Here are a few ways you can make your eating plan changes a little less jarring:

- Gradually increase the carbs you eat on low carb days.
- Add one high carb meal to the plan per day, keep it that way for a week, and then add another.
- Make sure you still maintain your calorie intake, so you're

eating enough food to keep you full, but not too much so you start gaining weight back.

- Instead of alternating high carb and low carb days, you could do two high carb days followed by a low one, then three and one, and so on.

Whether we like it or not, as humans, we are creatures of habit, and a few months of eating a certain way will "program" you to expect certain things. If you make a dramatic change to your eating, even if it's going back to more "normal" eating, you're going to have a tough time adjusting. So take it slow, work back towards your regular eating plan, and take time to acclimatize.

Watch for Changes

As you slowly wean yourself off your carb cycling diet, you may find that you have some unexpected side effects. An increase in carbs can cause all sorts of changes in your body. So it's a good idea to know what to expect, both so that you don't panic if you notice it and so that you can recognize that you might need to take your transition back to a more regular diet a little slower. These side effects can include:

- Sugar spikes and crashes. As we've already covered, when you eat more carbs than you probably should, your blood sugar can spike, but the spike is always followed by a crash. If you suddenly increase your carb intake, you might notice this happening. Try to keep combining carbs with a little protein and fat to smooth the curve and avoid the spike!
- Fatigue is a common side effect of the crash that follows too

many simple carbs. If you're weaning off a carb cycling diet and finding that you're more tired than usual, try carbs that are higher in fiber, so they take a little longer to digest.

- Bloating, gas, or digestive changes. Yes, unfortunately, our gut gets used to a certain kind of diet. When you change things dramatically over a short time, it can rebel! If you're weaning off a carb cycling diet, expect a little digestive discomfort, but if it's excessive, painful, or worrisome, visit your doctor to check if there are any other causes to worry about.
- Carb cravings are another common side effect of eating carbs. Unfortunately, there's a reason most comfort foods include carbs. Eating them makes us feel good, mentally, and physically. Be careful that you don't go overboard reintroducing more carbs and undo all your good work!
- Brain fog can also be a side effect of adding more carbs to your diet. So, if you're feeling a little slow, take it as a cue to get outside and get some fresh air, and slow down reintroducing the carbs.

It can and should take several weeks to go from one type of eating plan to another, and carb cycling is no different. Whatever the change you're making, you are bound to see some changes in your general health. If they are mild and manageable, give it a few days. You should see them reduce and disappear over time. Still, as always, if you notice dramatic changes in your health, you should seek medical advice.

Maintenance Eating for Carb Cycling

When you reach your goal weight or the "end" of your carb cycling program, you're not going to be completely starved, and you won't have spent months dreaming about doughnuts and toast. So, you won't be tempted to eat everything that stands still long enough. That's a great start!

But you will also need to make some changes to your eating habits to go from losing weight, to keeping your weight where you want it to be.

The key here is to switch from the total number of calories you need to lose weight to the number of calories you need to maintain it.

Back in Chapter 2, we looked at how we could calculate our BMR and adjust it according to our activity levels. Then, depending on our individual goals, we subtracted 250-500 calories to lose weight healthily. Now that you have reached your goal weight, you can adjust your plan to this maintenance level. Now that you have lost some weight and maybe gained some muscle, it will likely be different. Run through the formula mentioned in Chapter 2 again with your new figures, or use one of the other methods we discussed to find your maintenance calories.

This may take some trial and error and differ for every person. If you're unsure what it should be, you might need to speak to your doctor or a nutritionist to get their recommendation.

You won't need to be as strict about low and high carb days either. Still, you should always be mindful of the role carbs play in your body and how they contribute to blood sugar levels and fat storage. The most important part now is recognizing what your maintenance calories are and staying around that number.

While you won't need to completely cut out carbs, you should still aim to avoid highly processed and refined carbs and choose whole grains and wholegrain products, fruits, and vegetables instead. Make sure you're adding a little extra fat to your meals to fill you up, and always get enough protein.

If you do notice that the needle on the scale is creeping up, or your clothes are getting a little tighter, you can cut back a little on the carbs on alternating days again, until things are back in control.

The main premise of carb cycling, though, is to make sure you never have to starve yourself, and that by choosing the type of calories you eat, and when you eat them, you can stay in control of your weight.

Maintenance Exercise for Carb Cycling

When your intense carb cycling journey is over, and you've reached your goal weight, you're probably going to be a lot fitter than when you started. But, since you don't want to lose a lot of weight anymore, you need to make a few adjustments to your workout plans as well.

It's still a good idea to do a few higher intensity workouts per week and intersperse them with lower impact or strength training workshops. Still, you could probably also have a day or two off each week without it having too much of an effect on your weight.

If you do have more carbs or calories than you really should one day, consider adding a workout into the mix to bring everything back into balance. Remember that exercise is your secret weapon to regulate blood sugar and to control how your body uses the nutrients you eat.

Then again, if exercise makes you feel good, like it does for many people, it's perfectly okay to keep it as a daily part of your routine. If you notice you are losing too much weight, you can always consult your doctor or nutritionist and make some adjustments to your diet to keep everything in balance.

When to Switch Back

Once you've tried and succeeded with carb cycling, you've learned a skill that you can use to lose weight and get yourself into great shape whenever you need to. Because you are still eating well and getting all the nutrition you need, there's no limit on when you can use this plan, and because there are no special foods, pills, or potions required, you don't need to save up to use this plan. You can simply switch back from "normal" eating to carb cycling whenever you need to, and vice versa.

If you notice that you are starting to gain a little weight, or not paying as much attention to your eating and exercise habits, it's a good idea to plan a month or two of carb cycling to get everything back in balance.

As for how long you should stick to follow up carb cycling bouts, use your goal weight as a goal. When you reach it and are holding steady, it's time to go back to weaning off the plan and maintenance eating. But, as always, take it slow and gentle. Shocking your body with significant changes overnight is never fun, and even if it doesn't necessarily harm you, it can lead you to make unhealthy or unadvisable choices.

Balance Is Everything

As you can see from this section of the book, when you choose carb cycling as your weight loss and healthy living strategy, it really is all about balance.

When you eat a little too much of the wrong types of foods, you need to work out a little harder to balance it out. When you notice that you're losing a bit more weight than you would like, you can add a few more calories or scale back on workouts.

A healthy lifestyle and eating plan should never be about cutting something out entirely or about obsessing about every last thing you eat or do. Not only is that not sustainable, but it is also not healthy.

So, once you reach your goals, take it a little easier on yourself. Enjoy life a little more. Have a cheat meal once a week. And then make sure that you work out a couple of days a week.

The reason we don't stick to diets, and we find ourselves binging on everything we can lay our hands on is because we try to restrict ourselves too much and take an all or nothing approach. Carb cycling is all about an easier, gentler middle ground, and your lifestyle should be the same.

Eating is not all or nothing. You don't have to punish yourself if you slip, and you shouldn't be telling yourself you've failed anyway, so you might as well eat all the goodies!

Carb cycling is not a diet. It's a sensible approach to eating, limiting your intake of refined carbs when you don't need them and allows a little leeway when you do. It's all about balance.

YOU CAN'T CONTROL WHAT GOES ON OUTSIDE, BUT YOU <u>CAN</u> CONTROL WHAT GOES ON INSIDE.

Unknown

AFTERWORD

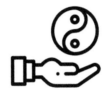

One of the biggest problems we face today is how to balance our busy lives and the demand for immediacy in our lives with being healthy.

We have less time than ever and more demands on us. So, we need to find easier ways to keep our health under control, and carb cycling is that for many people.

This is one of the few diet and exercise plans out there that don't require an all or nothing approach. You don't need to completely eliminate any single food group from your life, and it doesn't require you to devote your every waking minute to the plan.

Unlike most diet and exercise plans, you don't have to join a particular gym or buy expensive equipment. You also don't have to invest in ingredients you can't even pronounce or any celebrity-endorsed supplements. There are no special foods required, you can buy everything you need from the supermarket you always shop at, and you don't need any fancy fitness clothing or equipment.

You don't even have to tell anyone that you're doing carb cycling. If you plan get-togethers with friends for high carb days, you can even still enjoy pizza night or a trip to an Italian pasta palace.

While I can't tell you that it will absolutely work for you, and while it definitely demands commitment and hard work, it's a lot less restrictive and complicated than most of the diets out there. It doesn't require any expensive pills, potions or machines, and doesn't require you to artificially and impossibly restrict anything.

This is one of the most forgiving and easiest to manage eating and lifestyle plans out there, and provided you don't have any medical advice to the contrary, it's worth a try. In fact, many doctors and medical professionals recommend this type of diet to control blood sugar for certain conditions.

Most of all, though, carb cycling is easy to start, easy to stick to, and easy to incorporate into your life – even if you have a family and a busy job and life.

You have nothing to lose but the weight, and if you're tired of diets that are designed to fail, this can be the solution you were looking for.

HEALTH IS THE GREATEST GIFT.

Buddha

THANK YOU

Thank you for reading this book and allowing us to share our knowledge and experience with you.

If you've enjoyed this book, please let us know by leaving an Amazon rating and a brief review! It only takes about 30 seconds, and it helps us stand a chance against big publishing houses. It also helps other readers find my work!

Thank you for your time, and have an awesome day!

RESOURCES

We have used many resources to compile the information in this book. While we hope we've taught you enough about carb cycling to make getting and staying healthy easy, we know that you still might want to do a little more research. So, we have compiled a list of great carb cycling resources you can visit and read to find out more.

Effects of diet cycling on weight loss, fat loss and resting energy expenditure in women

https://www.ncbi.nlm.nih.gov/pmc/articles/PMC2951044/

Carb Cycling for Weight Loss

https://www.todaysdietitian.com/newarchives/0718p10.shtml

The Science of Carb Cycling: How It Works and How to Do It Right (2020)

https://legionathletics.com/carb-cycling/

Is Carb Cycling an Effective Eating Strategy?

https://www.verywellfit.com/is-carb-cycling-an-effective-dietary-approach-4175794

Blood sugars may be key to optimizing weight loss approaches

https://medicalxpress.com/news/2017-08-blood-sugars-key-optimizing-weight.html

Why do dieters regain weight?

https://www.apa.org/science/about/psa/2018/05/calorie-deprivation

OTHER BOOKS BY BRITTNEY & CRAIG

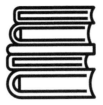

- Liver Detox & Cleanse
- Gut Detox & Cleanse

To find more of our books, simply search or click our names on

www.amazon.com

CPSIA information can be obtained
at www.ICGtesting.com
Printed in the USA
BVHW091547111121
621197BV00002B/271